Calling the Shots

Calling the Shots

Childhood Vaccination – One Family's Journey

Mary Alexander

Jessica Kingsley Publishers
London and New York

Contents

List of Tables

To Johnny, Jacob and Florence —
the best of families

Glossary of Terms

Auto-immune disease	When the body's immune system attacks the body itself.
CDC	Center for Disease Control – one of America's government-linked medical bodies.
Cochrane Collaboration	International organisation providing information on treatment effects.
CSM	Committee on Safety of Medicines – one of the many government-linked committees that monitors drug safety in the UK.
DOH	Department of Health (UK).
EEG	Electroencephalogram – measurement of brainwaves via electrodes attached to the skull.
FDA	Food and Drug Administration – America's drug-monitoring body.
Herd immunity	This occurs when the proportion of people immune to an infection is sufficiently high that transmission of the infection is very low. For a highly infectious viral disease like measles, this is around 95 per cent.
Immunisation	The process of introducing a substance into the body in order to provoke an immune response to that substance.
JCVI	Joint Committee on Vaccination and Immunisation – one of the UK government's medical advisory bodies.

'Killed' or inactivated vaccine	The disease element of the vaccine is neutralised or killed, meaning the vaccine is not infectious. Immunity conferred is generally shorter than with live vaccines. Boosters are required. Examples include Inactivated polio or wholecell whooping cough and tetanus.
Killed subunit vaccine	The vaccine consists of a small part of the disease element. An example is Hepatitis B and acellular whooping cough.
'Live' attenuated vaccine	The disease element of the vaccine is weakened but not killed, meaning that the vaccine is infectious. Vaccines containing live viruses or bacteria confer much longer immunity and have the highest levels of efficacy. Examples include the MMR and BCG.
MRC	Medical Research Council – one of the UK government's medical advisory bodies.
SIDS	Sudden infant death syndrome – also known as cot death.
Therapeutic medicine	Medicine given to someone who is already ill.
WHO	The World Health Organization.
Yellow-Card system	The way doctors in the UK report suspected adverse reactions to drugs.

Introduction

My interest in vaccination went from a 'normal' parental level to a possibly obsessive one in the space of 36 hours: the time it took for my small daughter, just two years old, to make the transition from a completely well child to a child suffering a serious, even life threatening, reaction to the meningitis C vaccine. Horrified by the hurricane which had hit our lives so unexpectedly, I went in search of information – first on the meningitis C vaccine, but inevitably this led me to wider, related areas: obviously, to the controversy surrounding the MMR jab, but also to the question marks hanging over other vaccines, levels of safety standards and the conflicts of interest that exist, to name just a few.

Some chapters in this book relate our experience as a family with the dark side of vaccination; these are interspersed with factual chapters that try to convey some of the information I stumbled across as a confused mother in search of some answers. I must make it clear that I have approached the question of vaccination not as a scientist or doctor (I am neither), but as a mother (which I am). As such, I've tried to ask the questions that mothers everywhere may be asking, and to look at the issues that really alarmed me when I received my vaccination wake-up call. I have endeavoured to shed as much light as possible on these areas, but acknowledge that, frustratingly, definitive answers are very often not available – even though in many cases, they undoubtedly should be, and with a little application, could be.

So this is not a vaccination book that advises parents on whether or not to immunise their child with a particular vaccine. That is a decision that lies with each and every parent. Instead, it is a book that aims to give parents information on some of the complex issues surrounding vaccination. From my research it seems to me that many of these issues – for example, the 'one size fits all' policy, and the ever increasing routine childhood vaccination schedule – need to be addressed if we are to continue as a nation to vaccinate our children with any confidence. Otherwise we may very well start failing in our duty to protect the youngest members of our society. Some scientists might say we already are.

Finally, I am very well aware how fortunate I am, not only to have Florence currently restored to full health, but also that I had the financial means to focus almost exclusively on looking for something that would help her, during her dark months of illness. I was able to afford to visit a range of private specialists when I felt frustrated by the shortcomings of the NHS; I was able to pay for tests that might reveal something useful; and I was also able to afford to visit a range of alternative practitioners. These, I know, are luxuries that many in similar or worse positions than I was, do not have access to. That they should is unquestionable; that they don't is an unpalatable truth in today's overburdened National Health Service.

Chapter One

The Question Mark over Vaccination

'First, do no harm' – Hippocrates

Over the last few years, vaccination has undergone a seismic shift in its placement in the world, from being a routine part of childhood to the stuff of regular headlines. Can the MMR (the triple jab for measles, mumps and rubella) cause a new regressive type of autism? Is the triple jab DTP (diphtheria, tetanus and pertussis) the cause of brain damage in some infants?

Behavioural problems now affect one in three children. Autism has apparently increased so dramatically across the developed world that it is now estimated that it affects one in every 150 children. Compared to 30 years ago, when the figures were more like one in a thousand, this represents nothing short of an epidemic. There have also been rises in a range of illnesses in children, including diabetes, asthma and cancer.

Vaccination, being a tool that directly targets and affects the functioning of our children's immune systems, has had the finger pointed in its direction on all of these counts and others besides. More and more people are starting to ask, are our heavy vaccination schedules playing a part in any or all of this?

HOW DID THIS vaccination confidence crisis begin? It really started with the MMR, which has been embroiled in controversy since the late 1990s. Despite steadfastly maintaining that the MMR is a very safe jab, the Department of Health has been unable to quash the uncertainty surrounding it. And so the alarm surrounding the triple jab has continued to sound.

Why has MMR uptake fallen to around 60 per cent in some areas of the UK, despite the Department of Health's repeatedly broadcast warnings of an imminent epidemic, and even a couple of isolated outbreaks of measles?

Why are so many parents taking their children's immunisation into their own hands, and seeking out single vaccines of measles, mumps and rubella, against the advice of the government, even though they have to pay for the privilege? Often they have to drive for several hours to find a doctor who will administer the jabs singly, but still they do it – making the round trip up to three times.

The willingness to go to such lengths can only imply a serious level of personal doubt in the safety of the MMR.

Why, although the government tells us the MMR is very safe, does the United States rate it as the second most dangerous vaccine behind DTP (which we give our children at two, three and four months)? In America, drug companies 'insure' against claims of damage by putting aside a small amount of money per vaccine they sell. This amount of money varies according to the risk associated with a vaccine. The payment is highest for DTP. Close behind it comes the MMR.

Question marks hanging over MMR may represent the starting point, but now the safety of many other vaccines is also being challenged.

Stories are surfacing of parents who fear their children have been brain-damaged by the DTP. One parent who is taking action on behalf of her brain-damaged son, told the *Daily Mail*: 'I am prepared to fight to show I am right. I won't always be around for [her son], and I want him to be properly looked after when I am not. Doctors have tried to tell me it [the DTP triple jab] was not responsible for what happened to him, but it was shortly after it that he began having fits.'

According to a report in the *Daily Mail* in autumn 2003, up to 120 families plan legal action against the vaccines manufacturer Glaxo Wellcome on similar grounds.

Why, in Britain, is the most widely used whooping cough vaccine the version that is well known by the medical community to be more dangerous than a more costly alternative? (For example, as reported in *The Scotsman*, February 2003, Scotland's deputy health minister admitted that the vaccine carried higher risks of adverse reaction compared with Infanrix, the DtaP alternative used routinely in the USA, Canada, Japan, Australia and South Korea.) A recent report compared the wholecell pertussis vaccine used in Britain in children as young as eight weeks, with the acellular pertussis vaccine routinely used in Europe, America and Australia. It was found that the efficacy of the two vaccines was the same, but the wholecell vaccine provoked 12 times the number of adverse reactions.

So why does Britain choose the more dangerous version? Can it really be for cost reasons? For the wholecell version's distinguishing factor, aside from its higher risk to children, is that it is cheaper to purchase.

The question has been asked, yet remains unanswered, whether there is a link between the pertussis vaccine and sudden infant death syndrome (SIDS), otherwise known as cot death.

The recently introduced meningitis C vaccine which the UK was practically the first country to adopt, has also had its share of controversy. On launch, claims were made that it had been rushed through trials, and some years on, while Ireland, Italy and Canada also now offer the vaccine, the rest of Europe, and America, a country which doesn't usually hang back on vaccinations, have not seen fit to put it on their schedules.

Then there's the growing concern over some of the ingredients contained in a vaccine, quite apart from the essential vaccinating components. Are these additional ingredients, often used to stop the vaccine going 'off', detrimental to our children's health?

In America, there are serious concerns over the effects of thimerosal, a form of mercury used in many vaccines since the 1930s. Thimerosal is very effective at killing bacteria and preventing bacterial contamination, but many parents question whether it is a possible cause of severe adverse reactions to some vaccines. Some, like those in the UK suing over perceived damage from DTP or MMR, are involved in long-running law suits claiming that thimerosal has damaged their children irrevocably. Alleged damage ranges from autism to seizures and stomach trouble.

While the US government has not admitted that thimerosal is dangerous, it has recommended that it be removed from future vaccines, and this is occurring. In the UK no such recommendation has been made, despite the fact that thimerosal appears in several children's vaccines, including DTP, given three times to a baby by the age of four months. Others are single tetanus shots and flu jabs.

Mercury is an acknowledged poison, so what is it doing in our children's vaccinations? In America, it has been calculated by a number of health organisations including the National Vaccine Program that infants who receive up to 15 mercury-containing vaccines by the age of six months may be exposed to dangerous amounts, amounts that exceed the safety levels that apply as set by the Food and Drug Administration, the body that monitors drug safety.

The addition of aluminium to vaccines, put in to provoke a greater immune response, has started to cause similar concerns. The

World Health Organization has responded by commissioning a scientific research body to look into the area.

Let's cast the net of worry surrounding vaccination even wider. Rises in auto-immune diseases like asthma, eczema and multiple sclerosis are signs that in increasing numbers of people, the immune system is malfunctioning. Something is causing this to happen, and vaccination is one obvious suspect. Are we, in our attempts to protect our children through extensive vaccination against an ever-growing range of diseases, actually causing them to develop other – often severe – problems instead?

Gulf War syndrome took some fit and healthy soldiers (with medical certificates to prove it) and put them in wheelchairs within a matter of months. Although exposure to radiation from shells has also been put forward as a possible cause for this dramatic change in health, many veterans pin the blame on the many vaccines they received in a very short space of time, before they were shipped out to war. Similar claims have been made by soldiers in America, who also underwent heavy vaccination schedules before flying out to the Gulf.

Regardless of the fact that this issue – whether giving many vaccines at once can cause significant harm to some – remains unresolved, the number of multiple jabs and the number of vaccines on our national schedules are both on the rise.

In America, many military personnel who received up to six compulsory anthrax vaccines have suffered appalling changes in their health, resulting in them leaving the forces. One such young woman went from being hailed by the military as one of the top pilots of her generation, at just 21, to being discharged a few years later in an appalling state of health months after having three anthrax injections. This woman now suffers from stiff joints, chronic fatigue, anaemia, memory loss, blackouts and permanent abdominal pains. Doubts about the safety of this vaccine are spreading, with up to 50 per cent of Britain's armed forces refusing to have this (voluntary in the UK) jab.

At the very time when more and more questions about the safety of vaccinations are being asked, so is public confidence in the government's answers in decline. People understandably struggle to believe in the government's answers when newspaper stories of large donations to the government coffers from drug companies with contracts to produce vaccines abound.

For example, according to a report in the *Daily Mail*, 2002, PowderJect, a company run by Labour donor Paul Drayson, was awarded a £32 million contract to produce a smallpox vaccine, just weeks after the second of two £50,000 donations was made by Drayson. Other companies tendering for the business, including Aventis Pasteur and GlaxoSmithKline, expressed surprise at how quickly the contract was awarded to PowderJect.

Equally, parental confidence in the judgement of their GPs is challenged when it is revealed that GPs are paid extra if they manage to vaccinate 90 per cent of their qualifying patients. Can a GP assess independently whether a child should have a vaccine or not, when he knows he is paid significantly more each year if he gives the jab? Such a policy has already led to abuse.

For example, some GPs have been reportedly so keen to have this bonus that they have, in the past, gone as far as actually removing from their lists those children whose parents wouldn't agree to giving the MMR. Thus they left only the immunised children on their lists, ensuring they still qualified for their bonus.

When it turns out that the committees that license vaccines for nationwide use often include people who also have strong financial links with the drug companies, levels of public confidence plummets even further. These links can include undertaking paid work for the drug cmpanies on vaccine related issues. Similar conflicts of interest exist in the United States.

And then there are the relatively fresh memories of the BSE experience. First, there were the government's repeated reassurances that BSE could not be passed via the food chain to humans, despite public concerns to the contrary. Eventually, the government had to admit that it was possible for people to contract CJD, the human version of BSE, through eating meat from infected cattle. This serves as a reminder to us all that the government can and does get it wrong, and that public health disasters do occur. Have the lessons from that public health nightmare (which is by no means certainly over) been learned?

AS PARENTS, WE need clarity if we are to vaccinate with confidence. The frightening reality is that nobody has the answers to many of these questions. As I have researched this book, I have heard the phrase 'nobody really knows' applied to the side effects of vaccination too often for comfort, everywhere from the corridors of the House of Lords to the plush consulting rooms of a respected paediatrician in Harley Street. This is a chilling acknowledgement of a routine feature of our children's lives, made by those amongst the very best placed to judge.

Despite this, it's not only natural for parents to want to get as close at it is possible to get to certainty on critical issues like this, but actually really vital, a responsibility that goes with parenting. All serious illness is sad and depressing, but there's something especially appalling about children being unwell. This is even more the case if that child is unwell as a result of a decision by the parent to give it something supposed to protect it.

Although certainty is very hard to offer – as one doctor said, the words 'never' and 'always' have no place in medicine – and although most people accept that all conventional medicine carries a small risk of side effects, and that includes vaccination, it seems imperative that the right questions are asked and the answers found, to make vaccination as safe a practice as possible.

Today's vaccination schedule

Routine vaccination is a feature of childhood in the 21st century, more so in developed countries but also in developing ones. Each country's vaccination schedule is based on an assessment of the diseases that pose a threat to the country's emerging population. Particularly in developing countries, what ends up on the schedule can be affected by the cost of a vaccine – some are more expensive than others.

One discovery made in the development of a variety of vaccines, was that they didn't always confer lifelong immunity, hence the need for several repeated shots of the same vaccine as a baby, and again as the baby becomes a child. This increases the number of vaccines a child receives quite dramatically to today's total.

Today's British child will receive 21 vaccines by the time it is 15 months old, and 29 by the age of five. At its first vaccine appointment at the age of two months, a British child receives DTP and Hib meningitis by one injection (a quadruple jab), plus at the same time meningitis C by injection, and polio, given orally. These are all repeated at three and four months. At 12 months, the MMR is given. The pre-school booster, consisting of oral polio, DTP, meningitis C and the MMR, is given somewhere between the ages of four and five.

In America, the childhood immunisation schedule varies slightly. There, babies receive hepatitis B at birth, and vaccinations of DTP, Hib and polio at two, four and six months, instead of two, three and four months as in the UK. At two and six months, the American baby also receives further hepatitis B shots. America uses acellular pertussis in the DTP, which is widely acknowledged to be safer than wholecell vaccines. America also uses the inactivated polio vaccine, where Britain uses the oral polio, which is a live version of the virus. At 12 to 15 months, the American child receives a fourth dose of Hib, as well as the MMR. At 15–18 months, they receive a fourth DTP shot, and a variacella vaccine (chickenpox) between 12 and 18 months. A pre-school booster, given somewhere between the ages of four and six, gives a child a further DTP, polio and MMR.

This means a fully inoculated American baby has received 26 vaccines by the age of 18 months and 33 by the time they go to school.

Australia follows America in its timing of the initial vaccines, inoculating at two, four and six months with DTP (acellular) and Hib, but giving polio orally. At 12 months, babies are given the MMR and Hib, and at 18 months a booster of DTP and Hib. A pre-school booster at four to five years of age includes DTP, oral polio and the MMR. This means by the age of 18 months a baby has received 23 vaccines, and 30 by the age of five.

In Canada, vaccination begins at two months, with DTP, IPV and Hib; these are given again at four and six months. At 12 months, a Canadian child receives MMR and meningitis C; at 18 months, DTP, IPV, Hib and MMR; and between four and six years, DTP and IPV.

This takes a Canadian child's total to 27 vaccines by 18 months, and 31 by the age of five.

Table 1.1 Childhood immunisation schedule – Australia

Age at which vaccine is given	Vaccine
2 months	DTPa; Hib; OPV
4 months	DTPa; Hib; OPV
6 months	DTPa; Hib; OPV
12 months	MMR; Hib
18 months	DTPa; Hib
Pre-school booster	DTPa; OPV; MMR
Total by school age:	30

Table 1.2 Childhood immunisation schedule – Canada

Age at which vaccine is given	Vaccine
2 months	DTP; IPV; Hib
4 months	DTP; IPV; Hib
6 months	DTP; IPV; Hib
12 months	MMR; Meningitis C
18 months	DTP; IPV; Hib; MMR
4–6 years	DTP; IPV
Total by school age:	31

Table 1.3 Childhood immunisation schedule – UK

Age at which vaccine is given	Vaccine
2 months	DTPw; Hib; Meningitis C; OPV
3 months	DTPw; Hib; Meningitis C; OPV
4 months	DTPw; Hib; Meningitis C; OPV
12–18 months	MMR
Pre-school booster	DTPa; Meningitis C; MMR; OPV
Total by school age:	29

Table 1.4 Childhood immunisation schedule – USA

Age at which vaccine is given	Vaccine
Birth	Hepatitis B
2 months	DTPa; Hib; IPV; Hepatitis B
4 months	DTPa; Hib; IPV
6 months	DTPa; Hib; IPV; Hepatitis B
12–15 months	Hib; MMR
15–18 months	DTPa
12–18 months	Variacella
Pre-school booster	DTPa; IPV; MMR
Total by school age:	33

Key to Immunisation Abbreviations

DTPa   diphtheria, tetanus and acellular pertussis vaccines

DTPw   diphtheria, tetanus and wholecell pertussis vaccines

Hib   haemophilus influenzae Type B

IPV   injected polio vaccine

MMR   measles, mumps and rubella vaccines

OPV   oral polio vaccine

Variacella   chickenpox vaccine

Chapter Two

Florence I

A Rude Awakening

The day that changed our lives was a colourless Thursday in early May. Looking back, I find I can't remember the date, or the exact weather conditions, which seems odd because I can remember all the details of what resulted from that day forward with crisp precision. But the part of the day before the critical moment that alerted me to my small daughter's dramatic change in health is largely lost in a hazy mental picture of a sea of such days swimming together to become one large picture representative of early motherhood.

Jacob was nearly four. Florence was just two. They probably woke me as usual around six thirty in the morning if it had been a good night, or I was already awake if it had been an interrupted one. Any mother knows that the joys of small children don't run to a full night's sleep being a Sure Thing.

Eventually, probably after a few well-aimed nudges with my foot – big toenail sharpened particularly for this purpose – against my unconscious husband's nearest shin had produced no results, I no doubt struggled out of bed and into a dressing gown, muttering darkly about the age of feminism having passed me by, and padded downstairs accompanied by two non-stop chattering children.

'Mummy, can we have pancakes?'

'No Jakey, want pasta!'

'You can't have pasta for breakfast Flo.' Two small bodies crunched up with helpless laughter as Florence begged for her favourite food three times a day.

Family life, going on in millions of households across the country. Cereal tipped into bowls ('Sorry darling, pancakes at the weekend I promise'), milk slopped in on the top, glasses of organic apple juice (must make sure they get their vitamins) doled out. Bread (wholemeal, organic) toasted, spread with butter and jam. A coffee for me, with hot milk, to encourage my brain to start to function.

Jacob must have been walked, I suspect protestingly, to nursery school. I'd over-mummied him, and now he never wanted to leave my side. I felt Maternal Guilt at every whinge, but I hadn't known you could love too much, only that a deficit produced known problems.

Maybe Florence went to the park that morning, or to the little music group in the local church. We had no appointments until that afternoon, when Jacob and Florence were both expected at our GP's surgery for their meningitis C inoculation.

Like most mothers, I had inoculated my children fully according to the routine childhood schedule. Like most mothers, I'd heard about the very occasional side effect. I didn't like vaccination days, but I'd always thought a combination of crossed fingers and a silent prayer to a largely neglected God would see me through. Mild side effects of fever and irritation we could cope with, and the more extreme ones, well, they were extremely rare, weren't they? As rare as being in a plane crash, and we took planes regularly.

Set against that slight risk were the known benefits of vaccination, and the scales tipped in favour. After all, polio, tetanus, diphtheria, whooping cough, these, along with the rest of the diseases that the vaccinations on the childhood immunisation schedule were designed to prevent, were serious illnesses, and it wasn't part of my child-rearing plan for my kids to get any or all of them. Vaccination was part of my culture – I even remember my mother ticking boxes on forms sent home from school ensuring I had a BCG jab, and also rubella – and had to be a Good Thing.

A nurse at the surgery gave both my children the meningitis C vaccine at around 3pm that day. The event was mildly traumatic. Jacob screamed and tried to brush the needle away, shouting 'Too pointy, too pointy' but to no avail. Florence just screamed.

Afterwards we went to get an ice-cream, by way of a cheer-up treat. Jacob licked his happily, and put the episode firmly behind him. But by the following morning, Florence was an unhappy child. She was flushed, clingy and miserable. She didn't want to be put down. I spent most of the day carrying her with me wherever I went, whatever I was doing. It seemed a dramatic change of health in a very short time: was it, I wondered, a side effect of the recently given vaccine? That afternoon, Friday, after Jacob had finished school, we all went to Bath, where we had just rented a cottage for the summer weekends. This was our second weekend there, and we didn't know the area well, although we loved its rurality and beauty.

That night, the cottage didn't seem such a good idea. Florence, miserable and hot, spent the night in our bed, restless and unable to settle. I lay awake most of the night, as fidgety as Flo, my hand repeatedly sneaking over to touch her forehead, or to poke the digital thermometer into her ear. I had a respect for fever in children, with both Jacob and Florence having had one febrile convulsion apiece in the past.

Febrile convulsions, the doctor had told me, were short, apparently harmless convulsions in children in response to fever, and were something some children seemed susceptible to but outgrew by the age of five, as the body matured and learned to cope with fever. Most children who were susceptible only had one, but occasionally, they might have a second before they reached the magic age of Five.

This information was at the forefront of my mind that night. The windows were open, we lay under a cool sheet, and Florence was on the maximum amount of Calpol and Nurofen. Occasionally, I cooled her down with a lukewarm flannel.

In the morning, gritty eyed from lack of sleep, my worry about Florence receded slightly as her temperature seemed so slight and she seemed happier. She ate some breakfast, always a sign of returning health in my children, and played with Jacob. She still returned to me for a cuddle more often than usual, but in the reassuring light of day I thought we'd seen the worst of this particular bug, whatever it was.

After an early lunch, feeling my lack of sleep, I crawled up to bed for a siesta. At first, Florence came with me, cuddling in, sucking her thumb, but she was too chatty and playful for sleep. After ten minutes, Johnny looked in on us and seeing her so restless and preventing me from sleeping, persuaded her to come downstairs to the sitting room.

The sitting room was directly beneath my bedroom, so when Johnny called my name a few minutes later, I heard him immediately. There was something in the quality of his call that had me out of bed in a second. As I ran down the stairs I was conscious of a force dragging inside me, a voice urging me to slow down, because once I reached Johnny and Florence my life might never be the same again. I didn't want to know what had happened, but still I couldn't get there quickly enough.

I turned into the sitting room doorway and saw Johnny cradling a greyish-blue, twitching, jerking Florence. I could see instantly that she was unconscious and convulsing.

'Call an ambulance,' I said to Johnny, trawling my mind for scraps of information from a recent first aid course and recalling that this was the first thing to ask someone else to do in an emergency. Johnny rushed off to the kitchen to the phone, while I laid our two-year-old daughter in the recovery position, and paused for a few seconds to give time for her breathing to restart spontaneously. I knew that if it didn't I would have to do it for her.

After a few more seconds, Florence took a shuddering gasp, and her face started to flood with colour. I allowed myself to breathe again too. 'Alright, darling' I crooned, even though it was far from alright, and my daughter, still unconscious, probably couldn't hear me. I was to find myself echoing this useless platitude too often in the next few months, seeking to give a reassurance I didn't have and couldn't find myself. It was not alright at all. Florence had just had a convulsion lasting a few minutes, and was still twitching away on the carpet, just as I could hear Johnny unable to tell the ambulance driver where we were. We were in the middle of some tiny hamlet several miles from Bath, and we had no idea how to direct someone to us. We'd only driven the route twice ourselves. Our minds blank with panic, we couldn't even recall the number of the nearest trunk road.

Unable to leave Florence, who was now breathing well but still unconscious and fitting, I couldn't help him, and yet I could hardly hold on another moment for the comfort of oxygen bottles and calm paramedics, who were undoubtedly better placed to save my child than me. We needed help and we needed it now.

I could dimly hear Johnny in the driveway, calling loudly for help, phone in hand. A brave and determined middle-aged female villager – after all, a strange six-foot-four man leaping about yelling for help must have cut quite a peculiar picture – stopped to help, and spoke directly to the ambulance men, giving directions. Minutes crawled by, and then finally, just when I thought I really had to cry, from the panic inside me winning the battle to push out the tears, they were there, two capable paramedics with their grass green crackly uniforms and their well-rehearsed smiles.

Soon Florence lay on the ambulance bunk with an oxygen mask over her face, now conscious and clearly terrified. So was I, but struggling to hide it. Why, I berated myself, wasn't I cool and reassuring, surely that was how mothers were supposed to react to this kind of crisis? I just wanted to burst into tears, for someone to comfort *me* and tell me it would all be alright. Clearly no one could, so I kept the tears inside and allowed the ambulance paramedic to tell me that contrary to my worst fears, this was nothing to do with the meningitis C vaccination but merely a febrile convulsion, oh, her second was it, well, I knew about them then, didn't I, that children did have these in response to a temperature sometimes. It wasn't that unusual to have a second, dear, in a child prone to them, she said. I really, really wanted to believe her, but I couldn't get that jab out of my mind.

Finally, we arrived at the local hospital, and were ushered into a cubicle that looked like something from a cottage hospital in a BBC wartime serial. There was a bed, and a thin cotton curtain in a predominantly green flowery print gave us a little privacy. Johnny, who had followed the ambulance in the car with Jacob, turned up moments later. He told me they'd been singing a song 'We're following the stripy ambulance, the ambulance, the ambulance ...', to try to normalise the event for Jacob. And for himself.

As fast as things had deteriorated, so they seemingly stabilised. Florence, now sitting up on the bed, seemed perky and chatty. The doctor who came to see us said that Florence had had a febrile convulsion, and that he was certain it had absolutely nothing to do with her meningitis C vaccine, but was just a coincidence in timing and probably the result of a viral infection. He examined her ears and throat, but unable to find anything, he told us that whatever it was had probably done its worst.

Febrile convulsions come at the start of an illness, he told me. You never have more than one with each illness, he told me. It is very important to keep her cool and well-dosed with Calpol and Nurofen, he told me. Sponge her with lukewarm water if the drugs aren't helping, he told me. And with that, we were free to take our daughter, still running a fever, home.

Thanking the doctor, I gathered up Florence in my arms and we left. Back in the car, Johnny and I gave each other reassuring glances. The doctor must know what he was talking about. Florence did seem to be getting better. She was chatting away with Jacob in the back, and kept saying she was hungry. It was getting late, long after their usual tea time. Perhaps this really was just another febrile convulsion, and nothing to do with the recent injection. Trying to bend my mind into the shape required to believe that, we got back to the rented cottage to find our friends, Neale and Deborah, waiting for us, confused but patient. In the chaos, we'd completely forgotten we'd asked them down for the night.

Coming downstairs after settling the children, I found Johnny in the back garden with Neale and Deborah, drinking glasses of icy white wine. I took a couple of huge gulps, feeling my shoulders up by my ears. I hadn't really had time to assimilate the day's events, yet at the same time, I was telling myself they were over.

'Relax,' Johnny told me, 'she's alright.'

But was she?

I couldn't relax. I telephoned my best friend Clare, and told her what had happened.

'I feel such a failure as a mother. It's as if I can't keep her cool. But I know about the risks of temperature, and I don't know what else I could have done.'

She sympathised and reassured, like good friends are meant to.

We went through the mechanics of a relaxed Saturday evening. We made some supper, and ate it at the long farmhouse kitchen table, the evening light poking its fingers through the windows. It was a really lovely cottage, built of soft Bath stone, with never-ending views from the back over planted fields. To one side of the house was a field that was home to several horses, and often they'd come and stick their heads over the wall that separated them from us, and eyeball us with their solemn velvety stare. Textbook stuff for the affluent middle-class weekending family eager to shake the urban dust and grind from their heels.

So why did I long to be at home in London, with the hospital where Florence was born just minutes away?

In a bid for peace of mind, something that was markedly absent that night, I went to bed straight after supper, settling down beside Florence who was in our bed. Her temperature was rising again, but there were two hours to go before she was able to have any more medication. I sponged her as she lay there, and her feverish little eyes stared up at me. I felt sure I could see fear there, or was that just the reflection of what was in my own eyes?

All night I soothed her and dosed her and waited for her to fall asleep, but she hardly did. Johnny found this to be too much nocturnal activity and he decamped to the spare room. I envied him that freedom, just to pick up his pillow and go, but equally I knew I couldn't swap places even if he offered. However bad it was with Florence – no sleep, constant anxiety – I couldn't be anywhere else. Times would come when I'd be blind with fatigue and Johnny would literally order me to sleep in the spare room, promising that he would look after Florence, but still I couldn't go. It wasn't that I didn't trust him to look after her. It was more that I needed to do it myself, and that need was ignited that night in that bed in our rented country cottage. It was then that my life-changing journey truly started. That of caring for a beloved, vulnerable child. A child

I had made vulnerable. For whatever the doctors said, I knew in the early morning light, as Florence started to convulse again, that these were not regular febrile convulsions. Instead, they were a reaction to the meningitis C jab. A jab I had chosen to give her.

'JOHNNY!' I YELLED. 'Johnny!'. This time it was my turn to sound the alarm. He stumbled in. 'Get dressed,' I said. 'Get Jacob dressed. We've got to go back to London.'

With a glance at the limp, twitching form of his small daughter, over which I was bent like a question mark, Johnny pulled on his clothes without a word. I could see from his face that yesterday's bravado – 'relax, she's fine' – had been just that. Like me, he had hoped this nightmare would go away, but had known in a dark corner of his heart that it wouldn't. You never get more than one febrile convulsion per illness, yesterday's doctor had said. It seemed we were in uncharted waters.

Florence had started breathing again, but this convulsion was proving longer than the last. Over five minutes so far and still, despite my willing it to stop, her limbs danced on. Her eyeballs were rolled back in her head and moaning, groaning noises were coming from her lips. I felt angry at my helplessness, uselessness, my inability to reach my child.

At least her colour was good, I told myself, stroking her forehead, and murmuring the meaningless 'It's alright, darling' over and over again. Finally the fit slowed and released Florence from its grip, like an iron fist slowly unfurling to reveal its crushed victim. What would I find? How changed would she be? Her breathing had started again fairly quickly, but any lack of oxygen could cause brain damage. She began to cry. She opened her eyes. She was clearly disoriented, but she knew me. 'Mummy,' she said, crying some more. How much did she know, I wondered, about what had happened to her? Where had she been in those terrible trembling, shaking five minutes? Was it like having a dream, was it that kind of unconsciousness? I hugged her close, seeking to reassure her despite my own fears.

I scrambled into last night's clothes. It was five o'clock in the morning. For once Johnny, a bit of a speed freak anyway, had a reason to drive like the clappers, and for once I, a cautious law-abiding driver, failed to nag him. Bath is a hundred miles from London. We were home in just over an hour. As Johnny drove, once again Florence rallied. She chatted and giggled with us and with Jacob, and Johnny and I sighed with relief each time she said something that made sense. Johnny couldn't help himself. 'Tell me the names of the Teletubbies, Flo' he'd say. He was only asking the question for both of us. When she correctly named the four larger-than-life creatures that were then taking the pre-nursery world by storm, we smiled at each other triumphantly. Her mind was all there. She was alright, had emerged seemingly unscathed. We were adults, weren't we, we told each other, powerful adults, and we would pit our wits against those convulsions in a bloodless battle and we were going to win. Whatever it was that was stalking Florence, it wasn't going to get her.

The fighting spirit surges easily enough, when you have a scrap of hope to indicate that your loved one might have turned a corner. It's when there's only bleak despair that it is hard to even dream of an eventual victorious return to normality. It wasn't some exalted state of living that we were asking, hoping, for, but just normal, regular, rather exhausting but rewarding family life with two small children.

We had an emergency 24-hour doctor number from our private GP's surgery. We'd recently signed up for this practice, in addition to our NHS surgery, which had given the meningitis C vaccination, because getting after-hours help on the NHS meant hours spent queuing at Casualty at our local hospital. We'd met the emergency doctor once, and when we rang on the way into London and explained what had happened, he said he would come at once. I also rang my father and stepmother and asked them to take Jacob for the day. Whatever the day held, I didn't want him to share any more of the drama. He was putting up a good front, but he'd already seen more than enough.

We arrived home just minutes before the doctor did. He examined a by now perky Florence, and we all made rather relieved jokes about how children always put on a display of rude health in front of the doctor to make their parents feel like over-anxious worriers who can't distinguish a cold from a life-threatening disease. Florence was certainly doing an award-winning version of this now, asking for a drink and chatting freely to the doctor. He said he couldn't find much wrong with her, but the inside of one ear was a little red. He recommended antibiotics to be on the safe side, and said that if she had another convulsion we should take her to hospital. Like the doctor in Bath, he reassured me about the meningitis C vaccine – nothing to do with it, he said. He wrote out the prescription for the antibiotics and gave it to a relieved Johnny, who was perking up once more and saying, 'Relax, darling, she's going to be fine.'

Grandma Marie arrived to collect Jacob, and was greeted with relief by all of us. Then a lot of things happened simultaneously in the space of just a few seconds. Florence climbed onto her Grandma's lap, sucking her thumb quietly. Johnny picked up the prescription from the kitchen counter, and said he'd go and get it made up at the 24-hour chemist now reinforcements were here. As soon as he'd finished his sentence, Marie asked, 'Is she alright, Mary?' and all eyes swivelled to Florence, just in time to watch her vanish in the grip of yet another convulsion.

I scooped her off Marie's lap and placed her on the sofa next door, trying not to absorb the fact that I was laying my small daughter in the recovery position for the third time in 18 hours. Fighting down the fast becoming familiar sensation of panic, I waited for the convulsion to stop, as it had the previous two times. For then, I knew, Florence would restart her breathing, her colour would return from grey-blue to a normal healthy pink, and the danger – of brain damage from lack of oxygen – would be largely past. I knelt at her side, stroking her back, helpless, willing her to come out of the grip of the fit, back to me, where I could reach her, care for her, protect her again. As a mother should.

'Come on, Flo,' I begged. 'Come on. You can do it.' But still the fit went on. Florence was very blue by now, and still the fit showed no signs of stopping, or even slowing. It was going on far too long. My mind divided. Half of it said, cry, scream, panic. The other half gave those thoughts a great shove and icily dictated, 'If she's not breathing, you need to resuscitate her. You know how, so get on with it.'

I held the back of Florence's head with one hand, and with the other pinched her small nostrils and lowered my mouth to hers. My lips were touching hers when she took a huge shuddering breath, hauling in the air.

'Well done, darling' I said, stroking her still trembling, twitching body, my own flooding with relief. All I had to do now was concentrate on her until the ambulance came. 'Well done, Flo darling, well done. It's alright, Mummy's here.'

It wasn't alright. It was very far from alright, and Mummy being there made little or no difference, but it was all the help I could offer her. What else could I say? My heart throbbed with love and my own sense of helplessness, my body stiff with fear. Please, God, I prayed – and I hadn't prayed since boarding school, where it had been compulsory – please, God, spare my daughter.

There is nothing so levelling as a mother's love, and I recall wondering then how many other mothers had knelt by their child's body, as I was doing, begging a much-neglected God for their lives? Millions of mothers in past centuries, more used to the agonies of burying their children but no less traumatised by doing so, as well as those from more recent times, closed ranks around me in my mind. Please, God, spare my daughter. Life without her was simply unthinkable. I prayed fervently. Dear God. Spare me Florence. I was truly scared for what was very probably the first time in my life.

Soon I heard the sirens, and then the ambulance crew were there. Calm and capable, utterly unruffled, they helped Florence, still convulsing but breathing independently, into the ambulance, and this time, with Jacob safely away with his shocked Grandma, Johnny followed us alone. Still I wanted to cry but knew I couldn't. Mustn't. I had to be strong, felt angry with myself for even considering crying as an option. I thought of my close girlfriends, my sisters-in-law, also mothers, and felt certain they wouldn't give way to the luxury of tears in my position.

What was it about me, that meant I always had to blub in a crisis?

The tears eased back to where they had come from behind my eyes. Florence was still convulsing as we arrived at the hospital.

'She's still fitting,' the ambulance crew said casually to the nurse in Casualty.

The maths was easy. That meant Florence had been convulsing for over 20 minutes. Textbook febrile convulsions, so a doctor had told me, were supposed to last less than five, and very rarely recurred within the frame of one illness. We had really chucked away the textbook now.

Florence lay on the bed in a cubicle in Casualty, Johnny and I standing beside her. A nurse popped her head round the curtain.

'Be with you shortly,' she smiled. 'D'you need anything?' The question felt faintly unbelievable. How about a healthy daughter?

Instead, I said, 'She's due for some more Calpol.'

'Oh,' said the nurse. 'Did you bring any?'

This was more unbelievable still. I knew the NHS was low on its resources, but I hadn't realised things had got so bad we were meant to supply our own medicines.

'No,' I replied.

The nurse returned, took Florence's temperature, dosed her with Calpol and made a note on her clipboard. Then she vanished behind the curtain once more.

There was a barely-controlled sense of emergency outside the cubicle but it wasn't about us. We could see through the gap in the curtain that several policemen were swarming about, and we heard mutterings about stab-wounds. Then I noticed blood seeping underneath the curtain separating our cubicle from the next. Some poor individual was losing a lot of blood, just feet away from us.

The cubicle on the other side of us suddenly began to emit panicky shouts. It turned out a crack cocaine addict lay within, thinking he was having a heart attack. We were so steeped in the details of our own crisis, yet we were just one of many confronting the yawning black abyss that was the uncertain future in this vision of hell. A place where only the desperate go.

An hour later, with Florence by now conscious, but listless, cuddled in my arms, a junior doctor arrived. Friendly and smiling, she asked for some details. I told her my by now well-rehearsed story, including the fact that this had begun with Florence's meningitis C vaccination. She was just the latest in a growing line of medical staff to dismiss any connection between the vaccine and Florence's illness.

She told us Florence needed to be admitted for observation, as the last convulsion had been dangerously long. She said she'd need to take some blood, at which Johnny, needle phobic, went pale and exited the cubicle. Easy for you, I thought furiously. It's Flo who's going to have to give it, and me who's going to have to hold her. But there was no time for anger, as there had been no time for tears. My energy had to be focused on getting Flo better.

Florence's hands and inner-elbow joints were covered in a local anaesthetic cream, and half an hour later the doctor returned to take the blood.

'You are a poor little chicken,' she said sympathetically to Florence.

'Am not chicken,' Florence returned crossly. 'Am little girl!'

The doctor and I laughed, and I felt my daughter was back with me once more. Being bolshy took energy and required mental power. I exhaled for what felt like the first time in hours.

But not for long. Finding a suitable vein proved difficult. Then, when the doctor finally got the line in despite a by now sobbing Florence's protestations, she dropped the first phial of blood and had to do it again. Finally, after a difficult 15 minutes, she had all the test tubes of shiny glutinous blood that she needed.

We now just had to wait for our transfer to the ward.

Meanwhile, the stab wound man in the cubicle next to us had bled to death, and the police were taking statements before drifting out. Florence expressed an encouraging desire to eat, so Johnny went out onto the streets of Paddington to look for yoghurts and fruit juice.

Eventually, after four hours in Casualty, we were admitted to a children's ward.

Florence had a bed in the middle of the ward, while I had a mattress on the floor. The ward seemed very full. Two separate areas contained toys, and there were several shelves of books. In one corner of the ward, a seven-year-old boy lay quietly in a wooden box that contained his whole body, leaving just his feet and head

poking out. It looked like he was part of a magician's act, about to
be sawn in half. It turned out he had lived there for most of his life,
going home very occasionally for a night here or there. As if to
heighten the sense of pathos, the box had been decorated with
stickers of the Teletubbies. Johnny and I exchanged glances.
Despite Florence's illness, we were clearly still much luckier than
some.

Day turned to evening, and the nurse told me that because
Florence had yet to be diagnosed with something, she couldn't
have antibiotics as this might mask the true cause of her illness. A
consultant came, and examined her, repeatedly pressing a blotchy
purple rash that had developed on both her arms. I mentioned the
meningitis C vaccine. He dismissed it, as I by now fully expected.
He made Florence move her neck and asked her several questions.
Was it stiff, he asked. He shone a light into her eyes. Did that upset
her, he asked. Florence wasn't sure. I knew he was checking her for
the classic signs of meningitis.

By nine that evening, Florence was exhausted. The ward was
noisy, with fathers pretending to visit their children but actually
watching the news on television with the volume up loud. I didn't
dare risk Hospital Rage by asking them to turn it down. I lay down
beside Florence and read her some stories. I longed for the familiar-
ity, the safety, the comfort, of home. I thought of Jacob, and
wondered how he was coping with all this disruption. I fantasised
about the Chinese take-away and glass of cold white wine I'd share
with Johnny when this was over. Possibly even this time tomorrow,
I thought, with a miraculously well Florence, tucked up in my bed
asleep.

During the night, there were two nurses in charge of what
seemed like about 40 children. I was the only parent I could see
staying the night. Just after midnight, Florence said her neck hurt. I
dragged a nurse over. The consultant stopped on his rounds and

checked her again. Still there were no answers. It seemed everything hinged on getting her blood tests back. What would they show?

Eventually, with Florence asleep again, I lay down on my mattress and shut my eyes. The next moment it was light. I'd slept in my clothes and felt like I'd been on a long-haul flight without the refreshing holiday part. When Florence woke up, we went to the bathroom together and cleaned our teeth. We had to wait for the consultant to do his rounds. Florence was still running a temperature, and I devoted all my energies to extracting her latest dose of Calpol from one of the busy nurses.

At 8am, Johnny turned up with Jacob, who was dressed for school. They brought coffee and croissants. Never had cappuccino tasted so good. Florence picked without interest at her pastry. Jacob jostled furiously with her for space on my lap.

The friendly paediatric doctor from yesterday morning's Casualty turned up to see how we were doing. She eyed the croissants longingly. I offered her one, which she devoured in seconds, telling me between mouthfuls that she'd been on duty since 6am on Sunday morning, and hadn't eaten since Sunday lunch. There simply hadn't been time. Having now worked for over 24 hours, she still didn't clock off until 6pm. I was shocked by the realisation that everything I had routinely read in the tabloids about the shortcomings of the NHS seemed to be true, and that my daughter's life lay in the hands of an extremely nice, but under-slept, under-fed, over-worked paediatrician.

But as it happened, it didn't. The paediatrician was called back to face another round of dramas in Casualty, and a new consultant came on the ward. We waited for his round like ardent royalists expecting a visit from the Queen. I suspect the sense of anticlimax was also similar. He glanced at his notes, then at me, ignoring Flo completely. He said brusquely that nothing seemed to be wrong with Florence, and that we could go home.

I was astonished. I'd repeatedly been told by various staff members we wouldn't be discharged until we had a diagnosis, and that that might not happen until the results of her blood tests came through.

'Even though she still has a temperature?' I asked, bewildered.

'Even though we haven't had the results of her blood tests?'

Much as I longed to go home, I didn't want to do so until Florence was getting better. I knew we'd just end up coming back again and every convulsion and ambulance ride piled up the trauma in varying degrees on every member of the family.

But now we were to be sent home. I would be given some leaflets on controlling temperature in children, he said. I felt as if he was telling me it was my fault. As if I hadn't bothered to administer Calpol and Nurofen, or sponge Florence to keep her cool. I glanced at the leaflets before mentally binning them. I had identical ones stuck up by the telephone in the playroom at home. They told me nothing new.

Johnny, who had left earlier to take Jacob to school, returned to collect us. With a feeling of unreality that was becoming familiar – was any of this happening, or had we made the whole thing up? – we left the hospital with Florence still undiagnosed despite three convulsions and a roaring temperature, and headed for home.

Once there, Florence settled on my bed. I rigged up a fan to keep the room cool, and sat with her, watching helplessly as her temperature started to spiral upwards. She couldn't have any more Calpol or Nurofen for almost two hours, so sponging and a fan creating a gentle breeze were my only weapons against the spectre of yet another temperature-produced convulsion.

After half an hour of watching her drifting in and out of consciousness, with my own mounting sense of panic and isolation, I called my private GP and explained the situation. Horrified that we had been let out of hospital without the test results, and with no reason behind Florence's three convulsions, he promised to be with us within the hour.

But I had no sooner put the phone down than it rang again. It was the hospital. Florence's tests were back. They showed that she had a streptococcus infection, coincidentally, so the caller told me, the bug that causes meningitis, although, she stressed, that didn't mean Florence had meningitis. But it did mean that she had to return to hospital immediately and start a course of intravenous antibiotics.

What happened if we didn't, I asked, fed up with the hospital by this stage and deciding I'd taken far too many of their statements in passive good faith. She might get septicemia and die, the caller replied. Why have we been allowed home, I asked in horror? It was a mistake, the caller admitted. The hospital was sorry.

I rang my GP back. He confirmed that streptococcus could be very serious, and recommended we return to hospital immediately.

So of course we did. Florence had to give several more phials of blood for further tests, and then was rigged up to a pump that pushed antibiotics into her via the line in her hand. The nurse told me firmly that although they were giving Florence the intravenous antibiotics used to treat meningitis, Florence definitely didn't have meningitis. Johnny and I glanced at each other. We later compared notes and found we were both thinking the same thing. Had the vaccine that Florence had been given four days earlier, the vaccine every single member of the medical staff we'd spoken to were so keen to dismiss, actually given Florence meningitis? After all, wasn't that how a vaccine worked? By giving a little of the disease, tricking the body into responding and thereby delivering immunity?

Much later, with a line in Florence's hand under a bandage in preparation for future doses of antibiotics, we were discharged for the second time that day. It was after 10pm, and the discharging nurse told me she had arranged for a home service visit each day to give Florence her IV dose of drugs. This, I learned gratefully, meant we didn't have to stay in for five days, or come back to the hospital each day for several hours. I knew this meant less trauma for all of us. We'd all had enough of blood and gore and children in misery.

Lying in bed that night, Florence by my side, her temperature finally going in the right direction, I reflected with astonishment that parts of the NHS could be so comprehensively successful – the ambulance service, the home care service we were now being offered, the quality of the majority of the individuals like the paediatrician with the impossible hours – and other parts – Casualty, the consultant who sent us home without waiting for Florence's test results, the way staff were so overworked – could be so dangerously below standard.

Every day that week, a charming nurse arrived in ordinary clothes – less alarming for Florence than yet another medical person in a uniform – to administer Florence's antibiotics intravenously. Every day we sat on the sofa, Flo and I, with Jacob close by, and watched cartoons on television while the drugs dripped into her system. By Friday – red letter day, the last day of treatment – it was impossible to believe that Florence had been as unwell as she had. I knew children recovered quickly, but still, I felt amazed. Amazed and grateful. My worst fears had been unfounded. The ultimate nightmare had not come true. Florence was seemingly alright, still the same little girl she had been before the whole drama had begun just a week before, albeit quieter and strangely disoriented.

It was a few days after Florence had finished her course of IV antibiotics, and was back in her own bed, that I finally got my

Chinese take-away and glass of wine, as fantasised about during all the dramas. As Johnny and I ate, we talked about what had happened to us all. We both wanted to believe it was over. That Florence was better, had been unlucky, had just had a bug and an unusual set of three febrile convulsions running together.

But I suspect neither of us really believed that. I went upstairs to my computer and turned it on. I was going to look up vaccination side effects on the internet, and see what information I could find. I needed to know where we stood with this experience, and whether we could truly consider it over.

Chapter Three

The History of Vaccination

Smallpox

The principle of vaccination – seeking protection from a disease by infecting a person with a mild version of it – has been around for a very long time. A thousand years ago, the Chinese were reportedly grinding up dried crusts of smallpox to the consistency of dust, which they then blew into a person's nose. This practice was called variolation, and several methods existed. Another method involved the introduction of material taken from smallpox crusts into scarified areas – open cuts – of the skin, most usually on the arm. Alternatively, smallpox material was introduced into an open vein. The hope with all these methods was the same: that the patient would have a mild form of the disease, and afterwards complete protection against it.

It wasn't until the early 18th century that variolation made its way to America, probably via an African slave, and to England, thanks to Lady Mary Wortley Montagu. Lady Mary was the wife of the British Ambassador to Turkey, where variolation was widely practised. She wrote enthusiastically about it in her letters, and submitted her own daughter to the practice.

With no reports to the contrary, I can only assume she survived. Some did not. Variolation, although not as dangerous as the natural disease itself, was far from perfect. It killed 2 per cent of people who underwent the process (while smallpox itself was variously estimated to kill between 10 and 30 per cent). It also had the significant drawback of leaving those who chose variolation contagious with smallpox for some weeks, thus potentially increasing the numbers of cases of smallpox, rather than the reverse.

Still, some people were willing to try it, and one such was Caroline, the Princess of Wales. In 1721, London was suffering from a smallpox epidemic and the Princess was desperate to protect her children from the disease, after one of them had very nearly died from it. But before she submitted her children to variolation, she first wanted some reassurance on the safety of this new (to England) idea.

With very different medical ethics prevailing then, a small trial commenced. Variolation was carried out on six condemned prisoners in Newgate Prison (they did at least volunteer). Five of the six went on to develop mild smallpox, from which they recovered. The sixth, who had already had smallpox, had no reaction.

The trial was deemed a success, the prisoners were pardoned, and Caroline, thus reassured on the safety front, presumably became a keen supporter of the practice. Nevertheless, she was in the minority, and smallpox was still responsible for one in ten of all deaths in 1770s London.

The 1790s saw the arrival of Edward Jenner on the scene, offering a more scientific approach to protection against smallpox with the introduction of his cowpox vaccination. This was ultimately to prove a huge turning point in the fortunes of the disease.

Jenner, a doctor based in Berkeley, Gloucestershire, had spent years mulling over the traditional country wisdom that milkmaids who caught the cowpox could not catch smallpox. Others had made this connection before him, but Jenner's great contribution to medicine was that he turned the theory into a practical preventive medical application.

Jenner performed his first inoculation – on James Phipps, his gardener's son – in 1796, by scratching his skin with metal infected with cowpox. When Phipps recovered from the cowpox, Jenner then tried to give him smallpox in the same manner, but James proved immune. He later tried to infect Phipps again, but still the boy remained immune.

As Jenner himself explained later in his paper 'The Origin of the Vaccine Inoculation':

> The first experiment was made upon a lad of the name of Phipps, in whose arm a little Vaccine Virus was inserted, taken from the hand of a young woman who had been accidentally infected by a cow. Notwithstanding the resemblance which the pustule, thus excited on the boy's arm, bore to varioulous inoculation, yet as the indisposition attending it was barely perceptible, I could scarcely persuade myself the patient was secure from the Small Pox. However, on his being inoculated some months afterwards, it proved that he was secure.

It seemed that this attempt at vaccination had worked. But Jenner had to work on for two more years before his discovery was considered sufficiently tested by the medical profession to permit widespread introduction.

One of the breakthroughs Jenner made during these two years was establishing a source of supply of inoculating material. To do this, he took infected matter from a person with cowpox, and passed it on to another person; he then took matter from that person, and passed it on to yet another. He effectively passed the original disease-causing material through five consecutive people in this way, before trying to infect the fifth with smallpox. But the fifth person was seemingly immune. Jenner had discovered that the

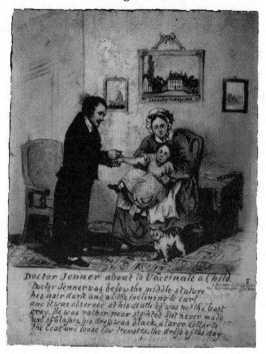

'Dr Jenner about to vaccinate a child'. Reproduced with permission of the Edward Jenner Museum.

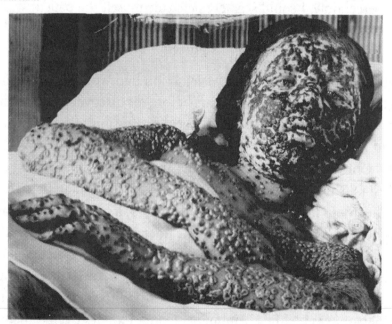

'A smallpox patient in the 1923 Gloucester epidemic'. Reproduced with permission of the Edward Jenner Museum.

The Vaccination Question.

A POPULAR

DEMONSTRATION

WILL BE HELD IN THE

CORN EXCHANGE, ANDOVER

(By permission of the Mayor),

On Wednesday next, Sept. 2nd,

TO COMMEMORATE THE RELEASE OF OUR

Heroic Towns-woman, Mrs. K. BLANCHARD,

Who has again suffered Imprisonment for refusing to submit her Children to
the WELL-KNOWN RISKS OF VACCINATION.

ADDRESSES

WILL BE GIVEN AND RESOLUTIONS MOVED BY

A. Milnes, Esq., M.A. (Lond.), F.S.S.

LIEUT.-GENERAL A. PHELPS,

and the

REV. W. C. MINIFIE.

(of Bournemouth),

Chair will be taken at 7.30 p.m. by Rev. J. HARPER

ADMISSION FREE—A few Reserved Chairs to avoid the crush, may be had at 6d. each
by previous application to the Hon. Secretary of the Andover Anti-Vaccination League.
F. R. Harvey, 78, High Street.

COLLECTION TO DEFRAY EXPENSES.

☞ The Reception Committee, Friends and Sympathizers will assemble at the
Town Station at 6.30 to Welcome Mrs. Blanchard, and will proceed from
thence to the Corn Exchange.

'Not everyone welcomed vaccination, as this poster illustrates'. Reproduced with permission of the Edward Jenner Museum.

protective element was retained each time it was passed on to another person.

In 1798, Jenner published his findings himself, and people began queuing for his inoculation. The process was grim by our standards today. Between two and five puncture wounds, depending on the practitioner, were made in the patient's hand or arm with small lancets, examples of which are on display at the Jenner Museum in Berkeley. (One can only hope that these rusty little penknives have not worn well with time.) The inoculating matter was then put into the wounds. Between days 1 and 15, the puncture marks would gradually turn black and swollen.

The risks to the patient included secondary infection, so the more puncture wounds a practitioner made, the more a person was at risk. Another problem was that the inoculating matter, taken from an individual with cowpox, might convey to the patient more than just protection against smallpox. If the person from whom the sample was taken had any other diseases, they could also be passed to the patient being inoculated. Syphilis was one disease that was frequently passed on to infants in this manner.

Despite this, to many people vaccination seemed much safer than the alternatives, and the practice began to become established. In 1802, the Duke of York had the entire British Army vaccinated. The same year, the government gave Jenner a grant of £10,000 in recognition of the significance of his work; and in 1807, a further grant of £20,000, to allow him to carry on with his work on vaccination without the distraction of having to make money to support himself.

Jenner, who had by now dedicated much of his working life to vaccination and would continue to do so until his death, set up a vaccination service in a hut in his garden – a place he dubbed the 'Temple of Vaccinia'. Here he inoculated the poor for free on specified days.

By 1831–35, due to increasing vaccination, smallpox deaths were down to one in a thousand. Vaccination was made free in 1840. In 1853, it was made compulsory for all children born after 1st August of that year, so laying the first stone in the establishment of the policy of routinely immunising children against disease.

But not everyone welcomed Jenner's invention, just as they hadn't welcomed variolation. Nor did many parents like the fact that they were told they had to do it. Many people just didn't want to submit their babies to the vaccine, and chose to pay a fine instead.

An anti-vaccination lobby quickly sprang up, claiming that vaccination didn't work, and that it could actually be detrimental to health. Those against vaccination included some members of the medical profession. Meetings, where prominent anti-vaccinators would make their case, were held across the country down the years. This opposition to the vaccine was bolstered initially by the fact that some doctors performed the practice badly, with contaminated or ineffective vaccines, or in smallpox hospitals, where the disease was rampant anyway and the inoculating sores in the arm were easy points of natural infection.

The overall result was that smallpox continued to circulate. It took a great smallpox epidemic in 1871–72, which killed 42,000 people across the country, to bring about a renewed push to stamp out the disease. A much more stringent system of compulsory vaccination was introduced, requiring everyone aged between 2 and 50 to have the vaccine. (Those who didn't want to were no longer allowed simply to pay a fine, but were prosecuted and fined, and were still expected to have the vaccine afterwards. If they did not, they were prosecuted and fined again, until they capitulated. It is an indication of how strongly some parents felt, that some were prosecuted several times during their lives. Some even had their household goods sold in marketplaces to pay the fine, and many who could not pay went to prison. Despite these heavy-handed tactics, many anti-vaccinators continued to maintain their right to refuse the jab, until finally a conscientious objector's clause was inserted in the Vaccination Acts toward the end of the 19th century).

At the same time, isolation hospitals were set up for those who contracted the disease. The practice of checking imported cargo for the disease also became routine. This focused onslaught, of widespread vaccination, together with the policy of containing the disease where it appeared, produced results. By 1898, 100 years after Jenner's original unveiling of vaccination, mortality from smallpox in London had fallen dramatically, to one in every 100,000 – less than 50 people a year.

Louis Pasteur

When Jenner was working on the smallpox vaccine, he was doing so, rather amazingly, without knowing how disease worked. He didn't know where disease came from, or how infection occurred. The prevailing theory at the time on the subject was that disease resulted from spontaneous generation. It was a French physicist and a chemist, called Louis Pasteur, who was responsible for the establishment of germ theory, which allowed future scientists to identify the germ that created each disease, so paving the way for the creation of many vaccines.

Pasteur discovered that airborne dust contained germs of primitive organisms, always ready to develop and spread if given the right opportunity. In 1878, he published his findings, and turned his attention to the study of immunisation against these diseases spread by germs. By 1879, he had discovered the process of attenuation – the practice of altering the make-up of a germ to reduce its virulence, while ensuring the germ still provoked an immunity response. Pasteur worked on to develop successful vaccines against anthrax and rabies.

It was Pasteur who coined the words vaccine and vaccination, from the Latin, *vacca*, for cow. This was in recognition of the work of Edward Jenner, who, with his discovery of the protection cowpox gave against smallpox, had, in Pasteur's opinion, produced a kind of attenuated vaccine.

Like Jenner, Pasteur demonstrated the efficacy of the rabies vaccine on an acquaintance. A young boy, Joseph Meister, was bitten by a rabid dog. His father brought him to Pasteur, who proceeded to inject Meister with his new rabies vaccine. The boy survived, and went on to work as the caretaker at the Pasteur Institute, founded in 1887. Meister certainly thought Pasteur had saved his life. Such was his loyalty to Pasteur that in 1940, he killed himself rather than admit the invading Nazis to the crypt where Pasteur was buried.

Pasteur also held a public demonstration to prove the efficacy of his anthrax vaccine. Cows, sheep and a goat, some of whom had been vaccinated against anthrax, were given a lethal dose of anthrax. The previously inoculated animals survived, while all the others died.

The Pasteur Institute was set up in Paris in 1888, and still exists today, a non-profit making foundation dedicated to microbiology, immunology and molecular biology. The development of new vaccines against disease is still a key function of the institute today.

Modern developments

What Jenner and Pasteur achieved between them was to tranform the life expectancy of millions of children. At the end of the 19th century, whooping cough, measles, diphtheria, polio and scarlet fever had a mythical monster's appetite for young children, and the younger the better.

And although improved nutrition and hygiene could go some way in protecting children from these diseases, and could help them come through some of these illnesses unscathed, there were still casualties amongst the wealthiest homes, as in the most deprived.

Examples of children lost to wealthy Victorians, who had access to the best living standards, abound. Emmeline Pankhurst, the suffragette, lost her first son Frank at the age of just four, to the childhood killer diphtheria in 1888. Such was her grief that she refused ever to speak of him again. Nor was this to be her only loss. In 1910, she lost her other son, Harry, to polio at the age of 19. Similarly, the writer Rudyard Kipling lost his seven-year-old daughter Josephine to whooping cough in the early 20th century.

In the years 1851–1890, infant mortality stood at 150 per 1000 across the country, a heartbreaking figure representing incalculable grief to thousands of parents. In London, and other cities, the figures were worse. The key child-killing diseases were to blame. High infant mortality rates were the norm, whatever one's circumstances. But could science deliver a solution?

It could, thanks to the discovery of the principles of vaccination by Jenner and Pasteur, and these principles still form the basis of modern vaccination today. The 20th century saw the rise of vaccination as a healthcare prevention tool, from one compulsory vaccine at the start of the century – smallpox – to the multiple vaccine child health schedules we have today.

Table 3.1 Approximate dates for the introduction of vaccines for general use

Year	Vaccine
1798	Smallpox
1885	Rabies
1897	Plague
1914	Tetanus
1927	BCG (tuberculosis)
1942	Diphtheria
1945	Pertussis
1955	Injectable polio vaccine (Salk)
1962	Oral polio vaccine (Sabin)
1964	Measles
1967	Mumps
1970	Rubella
1971	MMR
1981	Hepatitis B
1987	Hib Influenza
1995	Chickenpox
1999	Meningitis C

The basic principles of vaccination

First, the germ causing the disease must be identified. Then the germ must be treated – or attenuated – to ensure that it will not give the person being vaccinated the full-blown disease. This attenuation must be carried out always bearing in mind that the end product must still retain the ability to provoke an immunity response sufficient to confer protection against the disease. This is done in a number of ways, and the result is that there are several different types of vaccines. The three main types are live vaccines, inactivated (or killed) vaccines, and inactivated subunit vaccines.

LIVE VACCINES

A live vaccine is one where the disease element of the vaccine is weakened but not killed. This means the vaccine is infectious. The advantage of vaccines containing live viruses or bacteria is that they confer much longer immunity, quite often for life. Examples include the MMR triple jab and the BCG (tuberculosis).

Polio is the only live vaccine given routinely that leaves the patient contagious – that is, able to pass the disease on – for around three weeks after vaccination. (It is most likely to be passed on through a recently inoculated child's faeces, and this is why parents and carers must be vigilant washing their hands after changing nappies.) With all other live vaccines, it is estimated that the live element of the vaccine is so minuscule as to mean the recently inoculated are not able to infect others. As people with a weakened immune system are most at threat of the vaccine mutating back to the full strength disease, they are not given live vaccines.

INACTIVATED (OR KILLED) VACCINES

An inactivated vaccine is one where the disease-causing element of the vaccine is neutralised. This means the vaccine is not infectious. The appeal of these vaccines is that the germ cannot cause even a mild form of the disease it prevents, and can be given even to those with a compromised immunity. The drawback is that immunity conferred is generally shorter than with live vaccines. Boosters are required. Examples include the inactivated polio vaccine and the wholecell whooping cough vaccine.

INACTIVATED SUBUNIT VACCINE

An inactivated subunit vaccine is a vaccine that contains only part of the disease-causing element. This is another form of non-infectious vaccine. Again they are suitable for those with weakened immune systems, but several doses are required to confer immunity. Examples include hepatitis B and accellular whooping cough.

DIFFERENT COUNTRIES MAY use different brands of vaccine. For example, the Japanese used a different brand of MMR to Britain. Several brands of one type of vaccine can be in use at the same time in any country. This is because a government often commissions two or three pharmaceutical companies to manufacture the same vaccine, to meet demand. For example, Merck and Co., GlaxoSmithKline and Aventis Pasteur have all manufactured the MMR for British use. (One advantage of this is that if a vaccine has to be withdrawn on safety grounds, the country is not left entirely without a supply.) These vaccines will be designed to do the same job, but may vary in the smaller details, much as two brand names of, say, paracetemol may vary slightly.

The diseases and the vaccines

DIPHTHERIA

This is a severe bacterial infection of the throat and tonsils, spread through coughing, sneezing and saliva. The infection in the throat can develop into a tough membrane that impairs breathing, sometimes resulting in oxygen starvation. The bacteria also produce a toxin that, via the blood, affects the heart and nerves. Complications can include heart failure and paralysis of the limbs.

A vaccine was developed in the 1920s, using antibodies taken from a patient recovering from the disease. This vaccine was widely introduced in the 1940s. Vaccination has made this disease rare in countries like Britain where the vaccine is routinely given. Today's vaccine is inactivated.

WHOOPING COUGH

This is caused by a virus called *Bordetella pertussis*, with the major symptom being a persistent cough that can lead to coughing spasms that end with a 'whooping' sound. The disease usually starts with a mild cold, with the cough developing about a week later. Infants and children don't always have a 'whoop' with their cough. The disease lasts about six weeks.

Complications include encephalitis, the partial collapse of the lung causing permanent damage, convulsions as a result of oxygen deprivation, pneumonia and ruptured blood vessels in the eyes.

A vaccine was developed in the 1920s, but general use didn't begin until the mid-1940s. There are two types of vaccine, both inactivated: the wholecell pertussis, and acellular pertussis. The latter is well-known for provoking a lower incidence of side effects in patients than the wholecell, and was developed for this reason. In Britain, pertussis wholecell is routinely given to infants, while America, Canada and Australia, as well as much of Europe, opt for the acellular version.

TETANUS

Tetanus, commonly known as lockjaw, is caused by the spores of the *Clostridium tetani* organism, which lives in the soil. If this enters the body through a cut in the skin, it produces a poison that attacks the central nervous system. Spasms and paralysis can result. In the worst cases, a victim's bodily functions seize up, and they can waste slowly away.

The inactivated vaccine was produced in 1914; as a result, cases of tetanus are rarely seen in Britain.

The tetanus vaccine with those for diptheria and whooping cough make up the triple jab known as DTP.

TUBERCULOSIS

Tuberculosis (TB) is a disease that starts in the lungs following infection with the organism *Mycobacterium tuberculosis*. It is transmitted by close contact with those infected coughing up the bacteria. In healthy, well-nourished individuals, the body's defence mechanism can often eradicate the bacteria. Alternatively, the bacteria can lie dormant for months or years, reactivating when the person's resistance falls. The result can be a chronic cough, weight loss, night sweating, and a gradual decline in health.

Although the poor and malnourished were more at risk, the wealthy middle classes could and did die a slow, lingering death from TB. Prior to the development of a vaccine (and the discovery of antibiotics which are today used to treat TB sufferers), treatment consisted of rest and clean air.

In the 1920s, the BCG (bacille Calmette-Guérin), a live vaccine, was developed by the French scientists Calmette and Guérin, offering about 70 per cent protection against tuberculosis.

Today the disease is making something of a comeback. It is proving resistant to antibiotics, and work is ongoing on a more effective vaccine. It is those who live in the worst conditions – in the UK the homeless, for example – who are particularly vulnerable. London has rates of TB higher than those found in Delhi, and has been dubbed the TB capital of the world.

POLIO

Polio is caused by a virus that attacks the ends of nerves, resulting in paralysis in varying degrees of severity. Like smallpox, polio was not fussy in the choice of its victims. Sufferers came from all classes and lifestyles. Franklin D. Roosevelt, a past President of the United States, lost the use of both legs when he contracted the disease in 1921.

In the late 1970s, polio was still in evidence in developed countries. My matron at boarding school walked with one leg in an iron support cage, as a result of the disease. We could hear her approaching from far away, as her leg clunked heavily with each step. This gave us time to put the midnight feast away. To us, an early warning system of her impending arrival, but to her a painful and permanent legacy of the disease.

Despite Roosevelt's efforts to promote research into the disease – funding, then as now, was critical if advancements were to be made, but was often in short supply – it wasn't until the 1950s that a real breakthrough came.

Who discovered the polio virus? This seems a good example of how scientific discoveries can be the work of many men. John Enders, an American scientist who favoured tweed suits and bow ties, received the Nobel Prize for Medicine in 1954, for growing the polio virus in test tubes, a key piece of research in the battle against polio. But he did modestly maintain that 'no discovery in scientific work is due to the efforts of any one man, but always results from the work of many people'.

Meanwhile Jonas Salk, the American virologist also responsible for producing an influenza shot, developed a killed polio vaccine in 1952. To test the vaccine, one million US children were vaccinated with either the polio vaccine or a placebo. The trial was declared a success, and Salk's polio vaccine won great acclaim.

Great acclaim, that is, much to the fury of a Frenchman named Albert Sabin, who had also been working on a polio vaccine. Unlike Salk's killed vaccine, Sabin's was based on Pasteur's methods of vaccine production, of producing a live but 'crippled' or attenuated vaccine.

Sabin, who described Salk as a 'kitchen chemist … [who] never had an original idea in his life' had to be content with coming second in the history books. However, his polio vaccine was later adopted in conjunction with Salk's, and in some countries the Salk and Sabin vaccines are today given in alternate shots. Sabin's live vaccine carries with it the small but real risk of infection with the polio virus.

MEASLES

In 1954, John Enders, proving something of a star amongst scientists, also identified the measles virus, but it wasn't until the 1960s that a vaccine was finally introduced.

Measles is caused by a virus that attacks many organs in the body. The main symptoms are cold symptoms, a cough, irritated eyes and fever, with a rash appearing four days into the illness. After six days the symptoms start to subside and the child recovers. Complications include blindness, brain damage and death and, as with many diseases, are far more likely in malnourished people. In Third World children the death rate from measles is up to 15 per cent.

The vaccine is a live virus, and is now usually given in conjunction with mumps and rubella in the widely-used MMR.

RUBELLA

Rubella is a vaccine that children receive for the good of others, for the benefits of society as a whole. The disease is mild in the person who has it, so mild in fact that it can even pass undiagnosed, but it is dangerous for pregnant women, particularly in the first few months of pregnancy. The risk of damage to the unborn baby is high, and can include deafness, heart valve disease, eye problems and brain damage.

In 1962, one of Enders' colleagues, Thomas Weller, developed a rubella vaccine, although this didn't become widespread until 1970. The result is a significant decline in the number of babies born with congenital rubella.

The rubella vaccine is a live vaccine most commonly given as part of the MMR.

MUMPS

Mumps is caused by a virus which infects the salivary glands, causing swelling in the neck. The illness begins with fever, headache and fatigue. Then the salivary gland in front of the ear becomes swollen, and within one to six days, the illness has run its course. The condition can be so mild as to pass unnoticed. Infection of the testicles occurs more commonly in adults than children, but sterility following such an illness is extremely rare. Complications can occur if the virus moves to the brain, but again this is much more likely in adults than children.

In 1967, the Jeryl Lynn strain of the live mumps vaccine was introduced by Maurice Hillman, after he had obtained specimens from his own daughter, Jeryl Lynn, while she had the disease. However, no vaccine was introduced to the United Kingdom until 1988, when it was given to British children for the first time as part of the MMR.

The mumps vaccine has never been given routinely as a single injection in Britain.

MENINGITIS C

There are many kinds of meningitis, and vaccines do not exist against them all. Meningitis in children frequently starts with flu-like symptoms, including headache, fever, vomiting and fatigue. There may be a change in alertness, stiff neck and seizures. Meningitis onset can be rapid and the disease extremely serious.

Meningitis C is a strain of meningitis that particularly strikes young children and teenagers. An inactivated subunit vaccine was introduced in the UK in 1999 and government figures estimate that this has prevented 40 deaths a year. The USA and much of Europe do not give this vaccine on a routine basis.

HAEMOPHILUS INFLUENZA, OR HIB

This is another form of meningitis. Hib is a leading cause of bacterial meningitis, the most serious kind, that usually affects babies. A vaccine was introduced in the second half of the 1980s. This is an inactivated subunit vaccine.

CHICKENPOX

Chickenpox is caused by a virus. The illness begins after two to three weeks of incubation, with fever and aching. Tiny blisters appear after a few days, spreading in a matter of hours all over the body. After a week or so, the blisters scab over and eventually disappear. A child is infectious from just before the blisters appear until they are all crusted over. A common and generally uneventful childhood disease, rare complications include secondary infections of the skin and neurological disease.

A live vaccine against this well-known childhood disease is already given to children in America in conjunction with the MMR. Doctors announced in late 2002 that introducing the chickenpox jab to the UK is under consideration.

INFLUENZA

Influenza, commonly known as the flu, is an infectious illness caused by a number of viruses. Every few years a new strain emerges from the Far East and eventually arrives in Europe.

Large numbers of people catch influenza, and if they are otherwise healthy, they endure the symptoms – high fever, aching muscles, headaches, sore throat and a cough – for several days before generally making a full recovery. Those particularly at risk of developing serious complications like pneumonia, include the elderly, the very young, and those with existing medical conditions like diabetes, heart disease and chronic bronchitis.

The influenza vaccine was introduced in 1945, also the result of the work of Jonas Salk. This was a big breakthrough, as influenza spreads rapidly and epidemics could and did claim millions of lives. One of the most well known was the epidemic of 1919, which wiped out more lives in a matter of months as it swept viciously across Europe, than the First World War had done in four brutal years. Salk had been sponsored to develop the vaccine by the US Army, which needed a flu vaccine as soon as possible to help win the Second World War.

Vaccine types include an inactivated wholecell and a subunit version.

HEPATITIS B

Hepatitis is an inflammation of the liver, and many types exist. The glandular fever virus, for example, can cause a mild hepatitis. But some specific viruses cause a more severe type of hepatitis. Hepatitis viruses range from A to C. Some are acquired through chance, others, like B and C, through sexual contact.

Hepatitis B is usually acquired during adolescence or adulthood through sexual contact, intravenous drug use or occupational exposure. In the UK, healthcare workers who might be affected through exposure to contaminated blood, bodily fluids and needles, are given a killed subunit vaccine. But some countries, such as America, include this vaccine on their childhood vaccination schedule, giving the vaccine at birth. A vaccine was available by the early 1980s.

It is under consideration whether to give this vaccine routinely to children in Britain, following a rise in the number of cases of hepatitis B occurring in the British population.

Multiple jabs

In the latter years of the 20th century, multiple jabs made an appearance. The first was one injection for diphtheria, tetanus and pertussis, DTP, introduced in the UK in 1974; the second, introduced in the UK in 1988, was the combined measles, mumps and rubella vaccine. DTP-Hib is an example of a four-in-one jab.

The theory behind multiple jabs is that the number of visits to surgery can be kept to a minimum, so helping both parents, who have to take their child, and medical staff, who have to deliver the jabs. Trauma to the child is also reduced. Another key benefit cited is that the child also receives early and maximum protection against the diseases, rather than being left exposed as vaccines are given individually over a period of months.

In America, one example of four vaccines in one shot is MMR plus chickenpox. As scientists develop more vaccines to protect against more diseases, the view is that multiple jabs containing several vaccines in one shot, will become increasingly commonplace. Parents may be less keen. But as a paediatrician at St George's hospital in London outlined to a newspaper in November 2002: 'As we see the possibility of more combined vaccines becoming available, parents need to be advised as to their advantages as well as their theoretical risk.'

The global effects of vaccination

In 1980, it seemed that the ultimate goal in the war against one disease was attained, when it was declared that smallpox had been eradicated worldwide. By the mid-1990s, just two samples of smallpox officially remained, in laboratories in Russia and America. These were due to be destroyed in the late 1990s, but this was postponed, initially because scientists believed that the samples might throw light on other, newer, diseases, like AIDS.

Now, with the possibility of germ warfare heading the international agenda after the events of September 11th, America and Britain have both commissioned pharmaceutical companies to manufacture large stocks of smallpox vaccine. Britain ordered a minimum of 20 million doses from PowderJect. America has gone as far as inoculating some members of its population against the disease, including George Bush Junior, who apparently came through the procedure with no ill effects. However, with rumours that a rare and virulent strain of smallpox was in the hands of the Iraqis, there were some doubts about how effective these vaccines would be.

Other diseases are targets for worldwide eradication. The World Health Organization believes that polio, already eradicated in the USA, is just a few years off this goal. Measles, already erased from the Americas, has also been put forward as a target for eradication. But the achievement of this goal will inevitably have been delayed by the current confidence crisis in the MMR.

Vaccination scares and side effects

The current MMR scare is not a first for Britain's parents. From the very first introduction of vaccination back in the late 18th century, there have been sceptics, there have been critics, and there have been documented and acknowledged side effects. As we have seen, vaccines given in imperfect circumstances in Jenner's time, led to the belief that the vaccine didn't work.

More recently, a whooping cough scare in the late 1970s worried parents as much as the MMR does today. Then, parents were concerned that the pertussis element of the triple jab DTP, given at two, three and four months, caused brain damage in some children.

The scare, like the current MMR controversy, wouldn't go away. Despite government reassurances of its safety, several hundred parents maintained that their children had suffered brain damage as a result of the jab. The Vaccine Damage Payment Unit was eventually set up to deal with this crisis and some parents received small financial payments. The VDPU still exists today, although it was initially created as an 'interim' measure more than 20 years ago pending the introduction of a more satisfactory compensation scheme.

During the whooping cough vaccine scare, the government responded to parental fears by offering them a choice in the vaccination of their children. They could, if they wanted, choose to give their child the DT (diphtheria tetanus) without the P (pertussis) element over which the question mark hung. Pertussis could then be offered separately. (Today the three vaccines are once more given together.)

When the government failed to offer a similar choice for single measles vaccines in the MMR scare, parents were left to seek out the single vaccines themselves. This resulted in reports that the unlicensed single vaccines they were being offered were of questionable quality. Single-jab clinics were also criticised for seeking to profit from parents' uncertainty.

Today, as in the 1970s, much of the concern over the MMR vaccine centres on the possible overloading of a child's system by the giving of three vaccines at once.

Chapter Four

Florence II

The Damage Done

I sat in front of my computer and stared at the screen in front of me, struggling to absorb what I was reading. Apparently almost 5000 children had suffered adverse reactions to the meningitis C since it had been introduced nine months earlier. And an investigation had been launched into the deaths of eight children, to see if there was any link with the vaccine. Florence wasn't alone, it seemed.

Despite this, the deputy chief medical officer said that there were no plans to carry out a review into the safety of the vaccine. Instead, she claimed that the government was pleased with the initial results of the vaccination programme.

Over the last few days, I'd spent my scraps of spare time away from Florence on the internet, finding anything I could on vaccination. And there were only scraps of time available to me, because Florence was not the child she had been before her illness, so most of my time was spent with her. She was quieter and she tired easily. Her sleep was restless and her nights were always completed, if not begun, in our bed. In the day, her energy came in short 15- or 20-minute spurts, followed by long periods when she quietly tucked herself up on the sofa under a blanket and listened to stories or watched the Teletubbies, cuddling up to me, sucking her thumb. Unbearably, almost unnoticed at first, her strawberry blonde hair had started to fall out. She looked very pale. She wasn't ill exactly, but she certainly wasn't well. For a child supposed to be in the grip of the Terrible Twos, she was frighteningly good. From having been an outgoing toddler with a round of busy activities, she became instead my shadow, rarely seen far from my side.

But in those fragments of time, mostly in the evening when the children slept, I'd learned a few things about vaccination, including that the meningitis C vaccine was a new vaccine, and that the UK was practically alone in the world in considering it to be sufficiently well tested to bring into use. In other words, the children of the UK were guinea pigs for the rest of the world. If we didn't suffer undue adverse reactions, the rest of the world might consider using it.

So Florence, my Florence, my daughter who had just two months ago been photographed seemingly completely healthy celebrating her second birthday in a LaLa suit with a full head of hair, was now a mere statistic, if anyone cared to add her experience to their data and capitalise on it.

And that was a big if, because my friend Clare had already rung my GP and asked if there had been any adverse reactions reported to the meningitis C vaccine. 'None whatsoever' she had been told. Florence's experience had been miraculously airbrushed out of existence.

It was as if a policy of blanket denial could actually change events. If health professionals denied that there was any chance that Florence's illness had been related to the vaccine, eventually that would become the case. Certainly if the medics didn't acknowledge it in the first place, her experience certainly couldn't make it onto the Yellow Card system – the system that exists for monitoring reactions to medication – and be logged as an adverse reaction. Then the only person left maintaining that her illness had been caused by a jab was me, her mother, with no medical background whatsoever.

And yet, of course, Florence's reaction should have been logged. The Yellow Card system exists to report adverse reactions to drugs or vaccines, proven or otherwise. I didn't see how a child having three convulsions in the space of 18 hours, with the first convulsion starting just 36 hours after a vaccine, could not make it onto a Yellow Card on that basis. Florence's convulsions might not be a 'proven' reaction to the meningitis C, but it had to be a distinct possibility, given the timing. How could her experience be dismissed so confidently by every doctor I had encountered as 'Nothing to do with her meningitis C vaccine'?

Leaving proof aside, I just knew the jab and Florence's dramatic health decline were linked. I knew it as mothers do know things that concern their children, as they can. Doctors could deny the value of maternal instinct and crown science King, but mothers know their children, and a maternal instinct is something that other societies acknowledge even if we don't.

It was that instinct that had told me, from the first moment of Florence's first convulsion, that these were not straightforward febrile convulsions, as every doctor at every turn instructed me to believe, but an extreme and dangerous reaction to the meningitis C vaccine. I had witnessed both my children having a febrile convulsion once several months prior to the onset of Florence's illness, and both fits had been remarkably similar: alarming, but quick, over within half a minute, and the herald to a full recovery. Florence's convulsions following the injection had all been much more ferocious in intensity and ever-increasing in length. They had also marked just the start of her worsening health.

The irony was I would have loved to believe those doctors. I desperately wanted life to return to normal, to believe I had two healthy children again, and their diagnosis, however far-fetched, was far less worrying than my own secret fears. But I couldn't convince myself, because I knew it wasn't the case. I couldn't put the worry down. I couldn't tuck the anxiety away in a convenient fold of my mind and do as Johnny repeatedly exhorted me to do: get on with my life.

How I wished I could. I didn't want to think about it all the time, but if I tried to tell myself I was over-reacting, I only had to look at Florence to reconsider that point of view. Pretending nothing had happened to Florence, and that she was restored to health, was out of the question when she was so clearly not. In place of my previously thriving small child, I now had a listless, balding one.

The only way to achieve some peace of mind seemed to be through more information. I wanted information like a hippo wants mud. I wanted answers, something that would help me build a shield against the dragging sense of apprehension that never left me, that nagging sensation that something was nibbling at the pit of my stomach, a feeling that was there when I woke up even though I couldn't immediately remember what it was about, and a feeling that was all too good at stopping me getting to sleep at night. Fear.

Fear and I lived cheek-by-jowl that summer. It kept me awake, and when my exhaustion finally overcame it, it allowed me to sleep just a little, just enough to cope; while I did, it watched me like an ill-intentioned angel, determined to be there for my waking moment. The fear that this reaction to a vaccine hadn't run its course haunted me. Would it, like some monster from the deep, be back for more, for another bite at my daughter?

How could I be sure that the vaccine reaction was over? The fact that Florence now seemed so unwell without a particular cause seemed to imply it was not. Yet I desperately wanted to believe Florence was merely convalescing and would be back to her usual self in a matter of days. That way we could have some semblance of a normal life back.

I started to look for some more answers. I rang my paediatrician. I'd met him just a couple of times and he seemed likeable enough, although whenever I had tried to see him in the past he always seemed to be away on lecture tours. Sure enough, his secretary said he was away on yet another such tour, but that there was a very nice man called Ian Hay standing in for him. He could see Florence in a few days' time. I took the appointment.

Starting with a paediatrician seemed the most logical point of departure for me on my voyage for information and help for Florence. I was, after all, a conventional medicine girl, a fact perhaps best illustrated by the manner in which I'd given birth to my two children: epiduraled up to the hilt surrounded by the reassuring beeping of several machines and a bustling midwife in a blue hospital gown. I trusted conventional medicine, had chosen it over and above giving birth in a paddling pool while listening to Mozart. I wanted pain relief and medical expertise, not a lukewarm dip and a cup of herbal tea. That was the kind of person I was, the position from which I began motherhood, and the point of view I applied to the maintenance of my children's health.

It was this same culture of confidence in conventional medicine that had led me to follow the vaccination schedule outlined for children in the UK when Jacob was born. It had been a conscious choice to take up the benefits that conventional medicine could offer Jacob. When, a couple of years after Jacob was born, a friend told me she wasn't going to vaccinate her child, claiming vaccines didn't work and were bad for her child, I was sufficiently pro-vaccination to feel annoyed. I remembered thinking crossly, she's relying on the rest of us inoculating our children and sharing that slight risk of side effects, while her child remains safe from disease because of herd immunity, and safe from side effects, because she's not giving the vaccine. I left that particular cup of coffee convinced my friend was more selfish than I had previously realised.

So now, at a time of crisis, conventional medicne was my first port of call. The paediatric consulting rooms were concealed behind the elegant brick façade of what once would have been a central London town house. There were a few stone steps, the kind that posh men in top hats in *My Fair Lady* would have skipped up and down while singing. As I rang the doorbell, I was grateful I had BUPA health care, at the same time acknowledging that if I hadn't, I'd still have pawned my wedding ring to be here. I needed help, and hoped I was on the brink of finding some.

Ian Hay turned out to be a very charming South African man with a gentle but thorough manner and a consulting room full of toys. He listened to Florence's story as if it were the only story he'd ever been interested in his life. Afterwards he examined her, persuading her to co-operate with humour and patience presumably born of a long career working with children. Then he gave her a pile of interesting things to play with, and we sat down to discuss his findings.

He told me she'd obviously had a nasty time, but he thought it was unlikely to have been a reaction to the meningitis C vaccine. Although in this he concurred with all the doctors I'd previously seen, he didn't tell me, as so many of the others had, that the blame lay instead with my lack of ability, or lack of interest, in keeping my daughter cool. He said that he supposed that, occasionally, febrile convulsions could behave in this way, and that the length of the last fit left her worryingly open to brain damage due to lack of oxygen and must be avoided. This, he said, could be done through the use of diazepam suppositories which could be given rectally, if a convulsion lasted more than five minutes. This would bring the fit to an end. In the rare event it didn't, we could use a second one five minutes after that if the ambulance still hadn't arrived.

He also advised that if Florence had another convulsion, we should see a paediatric neurologist. To make sure there wasn't something else going on in Florence's brain. Like epilepsy.

I went home, and for the tenth time looked up Febrile Convulsion on the internet. This presented as a convulsion associated with fever in a child under five. I looked up Epilepsy. Unexplained brain activity leading to Grand Mal (complete convulsion) or Petit Mal (suddenly staring into the distance, immured from surroundings), cause not known.

Once again I found myself gazing at the screen in alarm. One of the more worrying things I was learning about conventional medicine was just how much the doctors didn't know. I'd imagined the term 'epilepsy' meant something more than an umbrella term under which to lump together all sorts of inexplicable brain activity resulting in convulsions. I'd imagined it was a condition caused by a shortage of something, or a crossed wire sending impulses down a dead end, which with medication could be corrected.

Instead, the approach was so much less specific than that, that all unusual brain activity that didn't fit in any other convenient category seemed to get filed under Epilepsy as if it were some kind of Miscellaneous file for all brain malfunction. I wondered how many fits Florence would have to have before she'd be moved to the broad 'don't really know what's happening' kind of diagnosis that seemed to be epilepsy, from the Febrile Convulsions pigeon-hole she was currently in. Febrile convulsion being, of course, a not dissimilar term for unexplainable convulsions in children under five as a result of fever that usually cause no harm ... Both epilepsy and febrile convulsions, I concluded, were essentially unexplained convulsions, that, a site on the internet told me, could be treated with sodium valporate ... the same drug for both conditions increased their similarites further.

I'D ALWAYS BEEN surprised the hospital hadn't arranged any follow-up assessment of Florence. In my quickly evaporating naivety, I'd thought that Florence's case warranted some kind of further assessment through the NHS. A few days after our appointment with Ian Hay, a letter arrived from the NHS, inviting Florence to an appointment with a paediatric neurologist. I didn't want to subject Florence to endless examinations – not surprisingly, her favourite game was now doctors and nurses with herself as the patient – but balanced against this was the fact that she so clearly wasn't well, and this would surely feed my appetite for facts.

Some weeks later, I duly took my pale, balding Florence along to this appointment. It took me a few minutes to realise that the paediatric neurologist, a small, dark woman in her fifties, and I had quite different agendas. I was after reassurance and help, but it seemed that she was apologising in an official capacity for Florence having been sent home from our local hospital all those weeks ago, prior to a diagnosis.

'Let me assure you that the consultant has been reprimanded' she told Johnny and me. We waved away her apologies, eager to get on to what mattered to us, namely Florence, only to find it almost impossible to deflect her. Johnny and I exchanged looks. We let her run her course. Once she had her apology out of the way – I wondered later if she thought that, American style, we were going to sue – she went on to tell us what we had come to expect from doctors.

That Florence's reaction was nothing to do with the meningitis C vaccination, but were simply febrile convulsions. Never mind that febrile convulsions didn't come in clusters of three in one illness, as Florence's had. Never mind that febrile convulsions didn't last 20 minutes, as Florence's last convulsion had. All this she waved away, together with the hospital diagnosis of streptococcus, the bug that causes meningitis. The test tube was probably contaminated by an external party, she said. Happens all the time, she said. No, Florence probably had a little viral infection, and it was just coincidence that she started to feel ill with this just hours after her meningitis C vaccine.

And some children, she went on firmly, did have convulsions that manifested themselves in this way, but parents could go a long way to controlling them if they simply made efforts to keep the child's fever down. This was the cue for her to pull out the usual 'Keep Your Child Cool' leaflets, which she promptly did.

At this the worm – me – turned sufficiently to refuse to take any more of these implicit criticisms of my seeming inability to dole out rather basic childhood medicines. 'I know how to medicate a fever, and I did all those things with Florence – the Calpol, the Nurofen, the lukewarm sponging – but still I couldn't prevent her convulsions,' I said. 'I kept a list at the back of my diary of the times I was giving her each one, just so I could be sure of not misremembering and missing a dose,' I said.

The paediatric neurologist looked at me thoughtfully for a moment, as if considering a number of possible responses. Eventually she replied with a sympathetic smile that perhaps I had applied these fever-reducing measures too energetically, and *that* had probably caused the convulsions.

I quietly disagreed with her. I told her that for whatever reason, it seemed to me that these measures, correctly applied, were simply not sufficient to control temperature in Florence. Was there anything else, I asked? Like Ian Hay, she prescribed rectal diazepam. It seemed this was to be the only new weapon in our armoury.

She then went on to spend a few minutes examining Florence, banging her knees and peering into her eyes before declaring that she seemed completely normal. Since she'd never met Florence when she had been what I would consider to be completely normal,

I assumed she was operating on a different scale of normality to me. But a balding, listless two-year-old who has previously been energetic with a full head of hair didn't immediately warrant a diagnosis of 'normal' to me.

We left, false smiles all round.

HOURS LATER, WITH Florence asleep downstairs, I sat in my study, my head literally resting in my hands. I had just had the worst phone call of my life.

During my evenings spent internet trawling, I had come across an organisation called JABS – Justice Awareness and Basic Support – a group that supplied information on vaccination. Today I had decided to ring their help line and talk to someone about Florence's experience, and see what their opinion was on it.

A man answered the phone. I explained what had happened to Florence following the meningitis C vaccine, and he told me that it sounded like a vaccine reaction. I asked him what might happen next, in his opinion. He thought for a moment. Then, he said, it can go one of two ways. Either, Florence would get better. Or, she would go the way of his son.

And what way is that, I asked.

It transpired that his son had started convulsing after the MMR. At first the convulsions were quite far apart in time, but gradually they had come closer and closer together, until now, several years later, their son was severely brain-damaged and having several convulsions a day.

The picture he painted was very, very bleak. And yet, having witnessed Florence's huge convulsions so recently, I could see her pitiful but relentless descent unfurling in my mind's eye like a silent movie.

'How long does it take until I know which way she's going,' I whispered.

Again, a thoughtful pause. Then, the verdict: 'If she doesn't have a convulsion for six months, you've probably got away with it.'

Got away with it! As if I'd taken some awful risk with my child's life, taken a gamble on her health, rather than taken her for a government-recommended vaccination.

Yet it seemed that was exactly what I had done. Because meningitis C was a new vaccine, and not part of the stable of long-established childhood vaccinations, where side effects had been monitored for some time, no one could say yet how a reaction to the meningitis C vaccine would manifest itself. All we could do was wait and see if the reaction had peaked and burned out, or if it was in its menacing infancy and would steadily worsen over time.

In other words, Florence could be on the road to recovery, or this could be the beginning of a slow and miserable slide into permanent ill-health and possible death. What the next six months held was, apparently, critical.

As I stared unseeingly at the white surface of my desk, I braced myself for what might be the hardest six months of my life. I anticipated a continuation of this state of living on my nerves, spending days and nights wondering whether Florence was about to convulse. Already I checked her several times a night, terrified she would have a convulsion without anyone there to help her. Already I found it impossible to leave her with anyone else in the day time. Except Johnny, but he was working all day. How could I? I'd never forgive myself if she had a convulsion and sustained some permanent damage *when I wasn't there.*

Not being there for Florence was unthinkable. I lived with enough guilt already – the guilt of having been the person who'd given her the injection in the first place – I didn't need any more.

We had to stick together, she and I, through the next six months, and face whatever was in store for us together.

Obviously this was going to affect how we lived our lives. Florence's most directly – for example, some of her little friends were gearing up to start nursery school in September, but how could Florence do that with such a massive question mark hanging over her future?

I imagined how cross Johnny would be with me, when I told him that I couldn't go out because I was too frightened to leave Flo. We lived in central London, and had a very nice and reliable babysitter the children adored who we had used frequently in the past, enabling us to do what parenting magazines told you is so important, to be a couple as well as parents, to see a movie, have dinner out with friends or just the two of us. But that was out of the question now. Because while it was fine to leave two healthy kids with a babysitter, leaving a child who might convulse at any moment with one was not. Who would be suitable to mind such a child – a paramedic crash team? I doubted they had time to take up babysitting opportunities.

It was clear our lives had to change to accommodate Florence, and to help get her well. That was a very small price to pay, if that was all that was demanded of us. I'd have settled for that in an instant. But it would take six convulsion-free months before we could exhale and shake hands with fate on the bottom line of this particular bill.

How could I have been so stupid? I asked myself as a fat tear plopped onto the desk. I had worked for several years as a journalist, research was meant to be second nature to me, so why hadn't I been aware that meningitis C was so new and untested that only the UK for some bizarre reason felt confident in introducing it?

I went back onto the internet and the more I read, the more self-condemning and terrified I became in equal parts. Here was all the information I had needed, had I bothered or thought to look. Posted on various health sites were letters from a range of people, including health professionals, explaining why they wouldn't give the meningitis C vaccine to their child; there was the story of a pharmacist who said she had no objections to vaccination per se but was refusing this one for her 11-year-old son as she knew it had been fast-tracked through testing and there were doubts about its safety. Another article outlined how a policy of vaccination might carry benefits, but children today were having far too many, often in one injection. The words I read matched the truth as I had known it in my heart, from the moment Florence started to fall ill following her injection. Why had I given her that jab?

THAT SUMMER, MY life became utterly centred on the home. I gave up the small amount of freelance work I had been doing, after finding myself attempting to write a fairly meaningless article at three in the morning. What was the point? I had to save my energies for a much more important job. Saving Florence.

I hardly dared leave her. My rare waking moments away from Florence were haunted by images of her convulsing, with no one knowing how to restart her breathing. At night, I had some terrible dreams. One particularly haunted me. It was a dark night, and Florence was missing. I knew, with a burning sense of urgency, that I only had a few minutes to find her, or she would be lost to me for ever. I was running along a badly lit London street calling her name repeatedly, only to hear it echo off into silence. My heart pounding in tandem with my running feet, I slowed down as I approached a builder's skip. Thinking Florence might be inside it, I started scrabbling around in it. I pulled off a piece of old, rain-dampened carpet, and found myself staring at a glassy-eyed Florence. I woke up and lay for what felt like minutes as still as a corpse, muscles frozen, lacking the courage to move.

Haunted at night, by day I was on a single minded mission to keep my daughter alive and well, to help her stay the person she was, and to ensure she had the future she deserved ahead of her. It was up to me – and only me – to make sure that she didn't have any more potentially brain-damaging fits. Whatever that took.

My hand would flit repeatedly to Florence's forehead several times a day, to check she was not getting hot. If in doubt, I'd give her Calpol. I knew this couldn't be good for her, and that she probably had it far too often, on a speculative basis, but if it held off a fit, wasn't that justified? I felt I was fighting a war against a force I couldn't see. I began to find bottles of Calpol everywhere – in the pocket of my coat, leaking into my handbag, in the glove box of the car. Equally distributed around our possessions were the Valium suppositories. There was one in the back of the buggy, another in the car, in my handbag, on the kitchen counter, in the bathroom. I marched to the beat of Just In Case.

The strain inevitably began to build. Johnny lived in the outside, busy, normal world, and Jacob spent part of each day at nursery, but I became increasingly homebound and tense.

Friends told me Florence looked well, that I should take a little time for myself, but I couldn't let go. I knew what they meant – that I was neurotic, paranoid, and had just got myself into a bit of a state over nothing. But what did they know? It wasn't their daughter who had had a series of terrifying convulsions. It wasn't their daughter who was part of a living trial. Some of them didn't even have children so how could they even begin to understand? I wouldn't have done, before I'd had children myself. I discounted all these opinions and continued to focus on Florence. If she looked a little flushed, I felt the flutterings of panic lick hungrily at my insides. If she didn't eat her tea, I held my breath to see what would happen next.

I really tried not to. I strove for a normal family front, for Jacob's sake as much as anyone's. At not quite four, my firstborn, my gorgeous blond boy, a tough little fellow who was also a Mummy's boy, was having to take a serious back seat in terms of his mother's attention. I strove to be fair, and tried to arrange to give him his own time with me. But Florence was just so much more needy, that that was where the bulk of my attention had to lie.

Jacob wasn't the only family member to feel neglected. Repeatedly, Johnny would urge me to get a babysitter, to go out, to see a movie. But I rarely did. I preferred to stay at home, just in case. Occasionally we'd go out for supper, to somewhere literally round the corner, within sprinting distance if the worst happened. Going to a film was unthinkable – after all I'd have to turn off my mobile phone. How could I relax if the babysitter couldn't reach me? What I was really most interested in doing was staying close to Florence, and counting: first the days, then the weeks, then finally, the months. We were slowly marching across the unmapped territory that was our critical six-month period.

Rare attempts at a social life often went awry. In June, I asked two friends round for a bowl of pasta. This somehow ballooned to six friends, who all knew each other. They just kept ringing, and saying 'Can we come?' and pathetically, I didn't feel able to say what I really wanted to say, which was 'No'. The dreaded night came round, and suddenly I found myself with a dinner party on my hands. Florence was listless – as she often was in that summer, so this was not a cause for alarm in itself – lying limp and hot on her bed upstairs. But once again instinct was hammering away inside me.

Something was wrong.

After greeting the guests – good friends, most of them – with a rictus smile on my face, handing them a glass of champagne and telling Johnny the food was in the oven, I then spent the rest of the evening upstairs, sitting on Florence's bed, wondering what the night held for her and me.

Every now and then, bursts of laughter would punctuate the low hum of conversation that drifted up from downstairs. Each time it did, I became even more tense. How could I nurse Florence effectively, lull her to a soothing, healing sleep, with that kind of racket going on? I crept downstairs and gestured to Johnny from the hallway, without the others seeing me. I asked him to get rid of the guests. He looked at me wearily. Was this really, truly necessary, he asked? I was immovable.

Ten minutes later, I watched from Florence's window as six people trudged out of our driveway carrying silver foil parcels – doggy bags. Although Johnny didn't agree with me, although he certainly thought I was an over-anxious mother on the verge of losing her grip on reality, he supported me then as always.

As it turned out, Florence's temperature hadn't been entirely in my mind. By midnight, she had a smattering of spots on her. By morning, she was covered. She had chickenpox. My mind could hardly compute this. Chickenpox, my family medical book told me, could be accompanied by several days of fever. Several days! It was like a life sentence. How would we navigate this without incident! Fever equalled convulsions in Florence's case, and these were inextricably linked in my mind too. I grimly engaged in the battle. I found a small notebook and started to record the amounts of Calpol and Nurofen I was giving Florence, and when, as if I were keeping accounts for a large and important corporation. In between doses, I stalked her with the digital thermometer. Large parts of each day were often spent splashing in a lukewarm bath together. Astonishingly, the days passed, the fever receded, and Florence's spots came and went without incident. She had had a fever, but no convulsion. I couldn't congratulate myself, it was far too soon for that, but I allowed myself to think that maybe, just maybe, we'd make it to our six-month deadline. The fact she could weather a bout of a childhood illness like chickenpox without a convulsion must be a good sign.

When I look back now at photographs of Florence that summer, I am surprised I didn't worry even more than I remember doing. Photographs taken in high summer show that she had just a few pale white wisps of hair left. Her eyes were quiet, her countenance passive. Her spirit was subdued, although certain things would excite her sufficiently to try to join in – she loved playing with her twin girl cousins, just a year older, when they visited from their home in Bermuda, and with Jacob. Her best friend was the second child of my friend Clare, a little boy slightly younger than her. That made up her social circle. While other children her age did the rounds of playgroups and playdates, Florence no longer had the energy for more.

Today that makes me sad, but at the time I was counting weeks and considering Florence to be doing rather well. I was focused on our six-month deadline, the deadline that the man at JABS had suggested might indicate Florence was not going to have any further complications from her meningitis C vaccine. This would fall towards the end of November. So I scrutinised Florence daily, tensed at the first cough and called our doctor if it lingered more than 24 hours.

All the rules I'd previously applied to family health – letting things run their course unless they were looking serious – went out the window. With Florence, every runny nose was potentially serious, and, as any mother can tell you, children have a lot of runny noses. We had a book on our shelves entitled *What to Do Before You Call the Doctor*. Johnny suggested we give it to the library, since it now sat neglected, gathering dust on the bookshelf, while my hand never seemed far from the receiver.

Our visiting 24-hour doctor, who saved us many a trip to casualty as so many illnesses seemed to strike at the weekend or at night, knew Florence's history well by now. We proceeded with caution, walking a tightrope: not wanting to neglect an illness that might cause a convulsion, yet not wanting to prescribe antibiotics in a knee-jerk way.

In August, we went again to the rented cottage in Bath for our summer holiday. We walked in the countryside, and swam at the local hotel's outdoor pool. My twin nieces came to stay, 15 months older than Florence. All four children ran about in the garden, with Florence desperately trying to keep up with them. When she couldn't, she'd dip her head and come over to me and put her head in my lap. I have pictures of her running up and down the lawn after her cousins, a pale wisp of a girl just leaving babyhood, confusion evident on her face. Why couldn't she keep up? The answer wasn't just because she was 15 months younger. She was struggling to do things against a fairly relentless tide of obvious exhaustion. Her cousins were kind to her, and took it in turns to play dolls with her while the other ran with Jacob.

On our last Sunday in Bath before returning to London, Johnny brought me a coffee in bed, and dropped *The Observer* on my lap. 'Meningitis advisers funded by drug firms'. The story revealed that four of the medical experts advising the government on whether the new meningitis C vaccine was safe had links to one or more of the drug companies that produced it.

Apparently, a member of the government's Committee on Safety of Medicines (CSM), had received support for academic research from US firms Wyeth and Chiron, who produce the two main meningitis products being used on children in Britain: Meningitec and Meninjugate.

Three members of the Joint Committee on Vaccination and Immunisation (JCVI) had also declared interests in vaccine manufacturers. One of them had served on an expert advisory panel for Wyeth, and received research grants from Wyeth and North American Vaccines, which produces a third meningitis C drug due to be introduced in 2000. Another had received funding from the drug industry to 'evaluate candidate meningicoccal vaccines'.

The secretary of state authorised the licence for the Wyeth vaccine, Meningitec, when the mass immunisation programme began in November 1999 on the advice of the CSM. The JCVI had also recommended the vaccine. Chiron, whose vaccine was introduced in April 2000, stood to make $200 million from the NHS deal.

Feeling like Anne from the Famous Five on the verge of discovering a seemingly nice relative is actually a mad scientist bent on creating some terrifying weapon of mass destruction, I looked at Johnny. So, there's big money to be had for drug companies if they can persuade the government to put their drug on the NHS childhood inoculations programme, I said. He nodded, and I read on.

The piece went on to say that in response to an article published the week previously by *The Observer* detailing how information on possible adverse reactions to the vaccines was being kept from parents, the chief medical officer insisted information on reactions to vaccinations would be sent, on request, to members of the public, health professionals or MPs, by the Medicines Control Agency (MCA). But the few readers who had tried this, had, it seemed, been unsuccessful.

Finally, details were given by the CSM and the JCVI of adverse reactions to the meningitis C. Apparently 16,527 adverse reactions had been reported including 12 deaths.

I dropped the paper onto my coffee cup. 12 deaths. It seemed we were one of the lucky ones. I snatched it up again and read on: Ah.

None of the deaths were found to be connected to the vaccine, the government said.

Then came the last blow. Apparently the figures detailing reactions were collated by the Medical Control Agency on the 'yellow card reporting scheme'. This, *The Observer* reminded me, was a scheme which requested health professionals to submit reports of reactions to drugs or vaccines, whether or not it was clear that a drug or vaccine caused it. The 12 deaths reported under this scheme might be an underestimation, since only around 15 per cent of GPs and healthcare professionals use the Yellow Card scheme.

Certainly my (former) NHS GP was among the majority 85 per cent who didn't bother. Which meant that *The Observer's* figures could represent just a very small slice of the true number of children reacting to this vaccine.

IN THE AUTUMN, Jacob went back to nursery school and Florence was once more at home with me. She was two and a half. Other children her age were going to nursery. Every morning when we dropped Jacob off, she asked why she couldn't go too. She said she didn't want to be the only baby at home. There were children her age at the nursery. And, as Johnny pointed out, I couldn't keep her at home on a speculative basis for ever. It wasn't fair for her to be held back by my anxiety. She had had a relatively good, incident-free summer. He urged me to try it.

With a complicated cocktail of fear and hope battling for supremacy in my heart, I agreed to three mornings a week. For two weeks it went well. I lived the life of a normal mother. For just a few mornings I walked both my children to nursery. Jacob was so happy his sister was going too, and kept informing me importantly of how he would look for her at break time and make sure she was alright. My boy with the great big heart had learnt quite a lot about responsibility in the last few tense months.

Florence, meanwhile, seemed to like it, and quickly developed a cast-iron passion for all things pink. She was, to my amazed delight, doing exactly what little girls should be: developing friendships, and her own preferences and opinions. Several times a day, I wondered if it was possible that she was really alright. After all, I could nearly touch November – it was now only a month away.

I began to relax. I remember telling a friend about Florence's progress, and joking that I wouldn't stop worrying until she was, oooh, thirty? Thirty-five? What I really meant was: 'I am starting to think, to believe, that there's a good chance she might be alright.' We'd had five convulsion-free months, after all. November was a mere hand's stretch away. Instead of an invalid convalescing on the sofa stalked by her mother with the digital thermometer, I had a little girl who went to the local Montessori nursery with her big brother a few times a week, a little girl who was making friends, learning to fly. I crossed my fingers and my toes. A girlfriend asked me to Paris for 24 hours at short notice. 'Go on,' Johnny urged. 'I'm here to look after the children, and it'll do you good.' I accepted.

A few days later, Florence began to cough. Not badly, just intermittently. By lunchtime, the cough hadn't disappeared but neither had it worsened. That afternoon, I described her cough to my GP over the phone, and we decided together it wasn't necessary to bring her in. It was, after all, just a cough, with no symptoms of distress or fever. Children had coughs and colds all the time. We'd monitor it, but at the moment, we decided to do nothing.

This decision was to become Serious Regret Number Two for me in the tale of Florence's ill-health. By relaxing slightly in the vigilance that many rightly or wrongly considered paranoid, I added to my already considerable guilt load. Perhaps, like a long-distance runner reaching the end of the field, I was worn out by the pace of anxiety I'd maintained during the last five months, and was flagging as I headed towards what I hoped would be the winning tape. Perhaps, as the Americans say, I just took my eye off the ball. Then there's always the possibility that, even if I'd taken her to the doctor, I wouldn't have been able to prevent what was coming. Whatever. 'What ifs' can go on for ever, but they don't change the result.

By midnight Florence was hot. Out came the notebook, in went the drugs. But all to no avail. At nearly 6am the following October morning, lying in my bed with Florence next to me, I heard the 'whoop' sound I had so come to dread. I started up into a sitting position and watched as Florence's eyeballs rolled back in her head, her limbs started to dance and her face twitched. She was having another convulsion. As Johnny telephoned an ambulance and shepherded a crying Jacob downstairs, I put Florence in the recovery position, stroked her head, tried to soothe her, although doctors had told me she couldn't hear me while she was fitting, murmured 'I love you, my darling girl, it's alright, mummy's here' over and over, all the while thinking how close we had come to November.

We'd come close. But we hadn't made it. So what did the vast black canyon that was the future yawning uncertainly in front of us now hold?

Chapter Five

Do We Really Need All These Vaccines?

The value of the vaccines we give today

In 1900, the world population was something approaching one billion people. Just a hundred years later, this figure had increased to six billion. This dramatic rise, unparalleled at any other time in world history, can be put down to two 19th century innovations: clean water, and vaccination.

Most people in their twenties or younger, have never seen anyone with measles. Who knows how diphtheria manifests itself? Most of us have never seen a case, let alone know anything about the membrane that can grow over the sufferer's airways, causing suffocation and possibly death, or the toxins that the disease produces, that slowly poisons the victim. Tetanus is largely a thing of the past, as is polio, which has almost been eradicated from the entire world. Clean water and good nutrition have helped, but vaccination has played an undoubted part in controlling these diseases.

But because we haven't seen these diseases, it can be tempting to think, well, maybe we don't have to immunise our children against them anymore. But unless a disease has been eradicated, the current general rule is that immunisation has to be kept up to prevent the disease coming back into circulation.

A good example of this can be seen by looking at what happened in an area that had a policy of country-wide vaccination, which was later allowed to lapse. In the USSR, children were routinely immunised against diphtheria and other childhood diseases. But with the break-up of the USSR, some immunisation schedules fell by the wayside, and outbreaks of diphtheria, amongst other diseases, occurred. In 1989, USSR reported 800 cases of diphtheria; by 1994, this had risen to 50,000 in countries within the former republic.

In the modern world, travel is fast and easy, providing easy opportunity for the spread of disease. Diphtheria may have started to regain its foothold in Russia, but the disease quickly capitalised on this initial stronghold and has now spread through several Eastern European countries. So it is argued that only immunisation protects our children from a disease that is hard to treat once acquired.

In the wake of the ongoing MMR scare, Britain is itself serving as an example of what happens when vaccination lapses. As take-up of MMR falls, so Britain has seen a rise in cases of measles. Figures from the Public Health Laboratory Service show there were 126 cases of measles in the first three months of 2002, compared with only 32 in the last quarter of 2001.

So just because a disease is not in immediate evidence does not mean it does not pose a threat. Immunisation must go on until a disease is eradicated from the worldwide population, or for ever in the case of bacterial diseases which are always present, such as tetanus.

Having said that, some diseases pose more of a threat than others. Diphtheria, for example, has very unpleasant symptoms and is hard to treat, while other childhood diseases, such as mumps, are generally much milder. Not so long ago, children would have routinely caught the milder diseases such as mumps and largely come through unscathed. But children have been immunised against diphtheria – an acknowledged killer – since the 1950s.

There was no vaccine for mumps in the UK until the MMR was introduced in 1988. This was despite the fact that the vaccine did exist and was used elsewhere. It was clearly not considered a vital vaccine that had to be on the UK schedule. Therefore most people my age had mumps as children and lived to tell the tale. Mumps was just something you had as a child in those days, in the way that today most British children have chickenpox, one of the rites-of-passage illnesses that parents accept as going with the territory of child rearing.

In the mid 20th century, mumps, along with some other childhood diseases like measles, was something that mothers actively wanted their children to catch, and would go to considerable lengths to ensure that they did.

Stories of measles and mumps parties in pre-immunisation days are common; mothers would take their children to tea with a friend's child who had the disease in the hope that their child would then catch it, on the basis that it was considered better to get the diseases over with in childhood. This would confer lifelong immunity, virtually guaranteeing that their children wouldn't have the disease as an adult, when, as everyone knew, they were much more severe.

But today we are told by the government that mumps and measles have very serious complications and that death can result even in the well-nourished middle-class child. The NHS website warns: 'Measles can be a very serious illness. There are often complications from measles and it can still kill.'

Certainly there is no doubt that measles can be a serious disease in some circumstances. In the Third World, measles accounts for three quarters of a million deaths each year. There, the measles vaccine can clearly save lives, and does so where the vaccine is given. But the Third World and the developed world are not comparable. In the Third World, malnutrition is the norm and the water supply often unclean, both factors that significantly impair health and resistance to disease. If a child is already weak from lack of good food and continual diarrhoea, thanks to a dubious water supply, resources to fight off a virus like measles are few.

In developed countries operating in an entirely different environment – that is, with clean water and good nutrition as standard – is the case for protection against measles different? Certainly the immune systems of the healthy well-fed British child should be functioning better and be largely distraction free – that is, not fighting another disease already – leaving it much better able to fight the disease and prevent complications occurring.

Dr Lockie, a leading British homeopath and qualified doctor, said: 'I had measles. My kids had measles. A healthy kid has a very good chance with measles, and is possibly better off as a result ... In the Third World, measles is a killer for kids who are malnourished. But so is everything else, if you haven't got the basics. It's a totally different environment.'

Dr Lockie believes that conventional vaccination is a good idea if it is well targeted. 'The homeopaths were there first on the theory of using the same thing to treat the illness.' (Having said that, Lockie doesn't believe that homeopathic vaccination works. 'All the evidence is that homeopathic vaccination alone doesn't do any good. If you've got someone who can't take orthodox immunisation, it won't do any harm, but I wouldn't rely on it.')

Is vaccination well targeted today? Our parents' generation had a handful of vaccinations, while our children currently receive 26 by the age of five. Increasing numbers of parents claim their children have been damaged by vaccines, rather than protected from a range of threatening diseases as is the intention. It is acknowledged even by the most conservative of medics that all vaccines carry at least a small risk of serious adverse reactions. There are others who would put the risk far higher.

And as Dr Richard Primavasi, a consultant paediatrician with his own private practice in Central London, told me in interview:

> The further down the field of vaccination we go, the less serious the diseases we treat. We started with smallpox, then diptheria, pertussis, polio and tetanus. Then it was measles, mumps, rubella, Hib and meningitis C. This second group are not such serious diseases as the primary immunisations. Therefore the health gain of these immunisations is not as great.

So could scaling back our current vaccination schedule to include only the diseases that pose a serious threat to our children be a possibility? The Department of Health (DoH) doesn't think so. A spokesperson for the DoH maintained that all the vaccines we currently give are neccessary. They said:

> People have forgotten what these diseases are like. Mumps, for example, was one of the biggest causes of viral meningitis in the under 15s. People could become quite ill with that. All of these diseases we used to see, they were part of the community understanding what these diseases were. Now they have gone, which is a really good thing. But as a consequence of protecting people, people now concentrate on the potential side effects and not on the dangers of the disease.

Compensation

The government is keen to promote the national vaccination schedule for children. But what help do they offer you if it goes wrong for your child?

Lord Ashley of Stoke has campaigned for compensation for vaccine-damaged children for 30 years, first as an MP in the House of Commons, and latterly in the House of Lords. He described vaccine-damaged people as 'the victims of a war fought on behalf of us all' and said they 'must be compensated for their sacrifice'.

The Vaccine Damage Payment Unit – note the use of the word 'payment' not 'compensation' – exists today thanks to Lord Ashley's efforts, amongst others. Payments for vaccine damage were introduced for the first time in 1979, when the Vaccine Damage Payment Unit was set up in response to many parental claims that the pertussis element of DTP had caused brain damage in their children. The conditions in which a payment could be made were very strict. The child had to be 80 per cent disabled by vaccine damage, and claims had to be made within a relatively short time limit.

Payment was a lump sum of £10,000. Given the tight criteria under which payouts were awarded, successful applications could be as few as just one in ten cases.

This payment system was meant to be an interim measure while a more structured form of compensating parents was devised. But 20 years later no alternative has been introduced by governments of any colour.

Under Blair's government, the one-off payment has been increased, first to £40,000 and more recently to £100,000. Time limits have been extended to allow more claims to qualify, and the changes applied retrospectively. The criterion of disability has been reduced from 80 to 60 per cent.

All of this is a step in the right direction, allowing more vaccine-damaged children to qualify for some financial assistance, but many consider it an inadequate system. Nobody could call a £100,000 payment compensation for the loss of, or severe damage to, one's child. 'This is not a compensation scheme,' said Lord

Ashley. 'Because it is so hard to prove that damage is caused by vaccination, the Government has a way of calling it a payment scheme, not a compensation scheme.'

There's no doubt that money helps hugely when caring for the sick. In my own experience, money (my own) meant, most importantly, that I could afford private treatments that otherwise would just not have been available to Florence.

Caring for a long-term ill person is an incredibly gruelling and exhausting task, draining the carer both physically and emotionally. Money means parents can provide a better level of care for their children, with slightly less stress to themselves and the rest of the family. Money means they don't have to work round the clock for the rest of their lives caring for their sick child. Money means a paid carer can share the workload with the parents and other relatives, and that means a semblance of ordinary family life can exist for any other children within the family.

There is also the issue of providing for a damaged child who might well outlive their parents. The current £100,000 won't go far in the way of lifetime planning.

Under the present scheme, the only real alternative that exists for parents seeking to provide fully for their child, is to tackle the drug companies themselves, as the 1000 parents suing over the MMR are in the process of doing. Everyone from the lawyers downward admits that this measure is a last resort.

America does it differently. There, vaccines are graded according to their risk, and the drug company that makes them donates a financial contribution per bottle sold, with the size of the contribution being determined on a sliding scale of risk posed. This results in a sizeable pool of money available to compensate those whose children are damaged by a vaccine. In terms of danger rating, DTP is seen as the most likely to cause a reaction with a levy of $4.56 per shot, followed closely by MMR at $4.44, polio at $0.29 and DT at $0.06.

This scheme was introduced in 1986 and means no parent is reduced to taking a pharmaceutical company to court as their only chance of receiving a suitable amount of redress.

Lord Clement-Jones, who has long campaigned for proper compensation to victims of vaccine damage, along American lines, told the House of Lords on 28 June 2000:

> If the Department of Health and the pharmaceutical companies do not take responsibility for past vaccine damage but hide behind the legalities of the law of tort and the requirement to show clear causation and negligence, it is hardly surprising that parents have second thoughts before arranging for their children to be vaccinated.

Big business and conflicted interests

Pharmaceutical companies have been criticised as being intent on one thing – increasing their profits. So just how big is the business of childhood immunisations in financial terms to companies like Merck, Pasteur and GlaxoSmithKline?

Clearly pharmaceutical companies are businesses, not charities, that need to operate at a profit. That's reasonable enough. And making a new vaccine isn't cheap. It can cost between $300 million and $800 million to get a vaccine developed and through the licensing procedure, the point at which it can be sold. That investment clearly has to be recovered.

Equally, there's no doubt that getting a vaccine on the routine immunisation schedule guarantees one thing: a constant level of sales, with a guaranteed supply of new consumers born each year. When the meningitis C vaccine was introduced, estimates put the value to Chiron, one of the pharmaceutical companies producing a vaccine, at $200 million per year. With those figures it doesn't take long to recoup $800 million development costs and be moving into significant profits.

A look at some company accounts reveals that vaccines do make serious amounts of money for pharmaceutical companies.

Taking GlaxoSmithKline as an example, vaccines earned the company £505 million in 2002. GlaxoSmithKline wrote in their half year review for 2002: '…vaccines showed strong growth worldwide of 13 per cent reflecting good performances in both the Hepatitis portfolio and Infanrix.' (Infanrix is DTPa, used in many countries worldwide to provide children with protection against diphtheria, tetanus and pertussis.)

Similarly, Merck generated $1022 million from vaccines in 2001, and says in its report that the 'MMR II, a pediatric vaccine for measles, mumps and rubella, Varivax, a live virus vaccine for the prevention of chickenpox, and Recombivax HB (Hepatitis B Vaccine recombinant) are the largest-selling…' [of Merck's vaccine products.]

Childhood vaccines are obviously of real worth to pharmaceutical companies. This fact sits uneasily alongside the knowledge that the government's medical committees – the committees that recommend new vaccines and monitor the safety of existing ones – include many individuals with financial links with the very drug companies that produce the vaccines.

Looking at a list of the members of the Committee on the Safety of Medicines (CSM) published by the CSM and available on the internet, valid from January 2002 to December 2004, for example, 18 of the 38 members listed had links with pharmaceutical companies, including research funding, grants, non-executive directorships and shares. The CSM is a powerful committee that can recommend to the government whether to license a new drug. It also monitors the safety of medicines once licensed and carries out reviews periodically on new medicines that might be causing concern.

Nor is the Medical Research Council (MCR), another influential government funded body, exempt from possible conflicts of interest. An article in *The Telegraph* in 2002 said 'The...Medical Research Committee, which decided that no further research was needed into the links between MMR and autism, included three members (out of 14) who are paid consultants for the vaccine manufacturers in the forthcoming legal case'. *The Telegraph* went on to add that the committee's chairman was also a GlaxoSmithKline shareholder (one of the drug companies involved in the MMR case).

The Joint Committee on Vaccination and Immunisation (JCVI), which advises the government on diseases preventable through vaccination, amongst other things, is well populated by individals with wide-ranging and current financial links with Merck, GlaxoSmithKline and Wyeth, amongst others. The declaration of interest statement for members of the JCVI, as published on the internet in late 2002, appears equally well-populated with individuals with wide-ranging links with the vaccine-producing drug companies including GlaxoSmithKline, Wyeth and Aventis Pasteur; others work in departments funded at least in part by drug companies; others carry out research into various aspects of vaccine safety and efficacy, funded once again by the relevant drug company.

Meningitis C, the vaccine that made my daughter so ill, also has some history in terms of potentially conflicting relationships between medical experts advising the government to adopt the vaccine, and the links these experts have with the drug companies that produce it. One of the members on the Medical Research Council had links with one of the companies producing a meningitis C vaccine, as did three of those on the JCVI. The chairmen of each of these committees issued statements reassuring the public on the safety of the vaccine after a newspaper reported thousands of adverse reactions amongst patients, including 12 deaths.

It was on advice from both of these committees that the vaccine was licensed by the secretary of state in the first place.

It is very possible that there is absolutely nothing of concern about any of this – other than the appearance of the thing. Clearly medical advisory committees do need contributions from experts with relevant experience. Nor are such issues exclusive to Britain.

In America, the committee on Government Reform was set up to examine conflict of interest and vaccine development. It found very similar conflicts of interest.

This report, published in August 2002, focused on two influential advisory committees used by federal regulators to provide expert advice on vaccine policy. These were the Food and Drug Administration's (FDA) Vaccines and Related Biological Products Advisory Committee (VRBPAC), and the Centers for Disease Control's (CDC) Advisory Committee on Immunisation Practices (ACIP). The report found that

> conflict of interest rules employed by the FDA and the CDC have been weak, enforcement has been lax, and committee members with substantial ties to pharmaceutical companies have been given waivers to participate in committee proceedings.

Among specific problems noted were the CDC routinely granting waivers from conflict of interest rules to every member of its advisory committee; CDC members who were not allowed to vote on certain recommendations due to financial conflicts of interest were still allowed to participate in committee deliberations and advocate specific positions; the chairman of the CDC's advisory committee had until recently owned 600 shares in Merck, a pharmaceutical company with an active vaccine division; members of the CDC's advisory committee often left key details out of their financial disclosure statements, and were not required to provide the missing information by CDC ethics officials.

While nothing is done to alter this current state of affairs, situations that illustrate how the present structure can lead to problems will continue to arise. One such is as follows. In 2002, the Medicines Control Agency (MCA), yet another of the UK government's medical committees, was asked to investigate a contraceptive pill, which Dr Joe Collier, editor of *Drug and Therapeutics Bulletin*, had pointed out was being promoted with claims that he felt the pill did not deliver. The MCA initially cleared the pill of any misrepresentation, and the company that produced it prepared to sue the doctor who had raised the alarm. Dr Collier refused to back down, and eventually the MCA had to revisit the issue, this time substantiating the doctor's view that the drug claimed to do something it did not achieve.

Dr Collier went on to tell *The Observer* (8 December 2002):

> There should be a full inquiry into how the MCA, which is partly funded by the pharmaceutical industry, allowed this advert to go through. This level of incompetence, which would appear to favour the industry rather than public health, is totally unacceptable.

GPs and performance-related pay

There's also a conflict of interest issue with the structuring of the pay of GPs. Effectively, GPs get paid more if they manage to immunise more than 90 per cent of the children on their lists with the appropriate vaccination. This kind of performance-related pay is all very well if you are in the double-glazing industry but is it really appropriate in medicine?

GPs generally have a huge commitment to the health of the patients in their care and would very probably not decide to immunise a child on the strength of a financial incentive rather than for the child's perceived health benefits. But what this system allows is for this doubt to exist in the parents mind, so undermining the essential element of trust between the parent and the doctor, and by extension, the parent and the government's recommended immunisation schedule.

A spokesperson at the Department of Health maintained that this issue was one of possibly deliberate misunderstanding:

> It's all [a] question of how people choose to portray it. If you are looking for a negative representation, it's quite easy to find. My understanding of the GP payment system is that a GP's salary is composed of various bits, and the vaccine target payments are just one of those bits. So basically they're being paid for doing good work ... if they don't do the work, they don't get the money ... it's not additional money, it's part of their income, but they have to perform in order to get it.

Nevertheless, the Department of Health admitted that 'at 70 per cent (of inoculated population) they get the baseline, if they achieve 90 per cent they get more'.

It's a fine distinction that some obviously miss. Certainly one doctor felt concerned enough about the potential for the public to perceive this as a conflict of interest to raise the subject at the British Medical Association's conference in summer 2002, recommending that the system worked against GPs and that it should be rethought.

And as we have already seen, such a pay system has already resulted in some GPs removing patients who won't have the MMR from their lists, in order to qualify for their bonus.

Independence of judgment must be rather like justice. It is a fundamental tenet of the law that the responsibility of a court system is not only that justice is done, but also that it is *seen* to be done. As a rule, judges don't sit on any case where they may have any per-ceived conflict of interest. This reflects the fact that the public must have confidence in the administration of justice, that is, the deci-sions judges reach. The same level of confidence seems necessary in health areas. When the government's medical committees pro-nounce a vaccine to be safe, or otherwise, the public must be able to have confidence in the unbiased truth of that statement.

Chapter Six

Florence III

Strains, Planes and Ambulance Rides

Once more Florence and I were taking an ambulance ride to the hospital. Florence had stopped convulsing, and was sitting whimpering and confused, strapped on the bed, wrapped in my arms, as the ambulance weaved its way through London's early morning traffic.

This time, while Johnny had called the ambulance and looked after a bewildered Jacob, I'd actually managed to pack a bag while watching the unconscious but no longer fitting Florence. I'd even included my own Calpol. I was learning. But what a learning curve. Mother coping with repeatedly ill child. It wasn't one I'd ever aspired to climb. I could barely believe it was me coping sometimes, it was almost like watching someone else. I lived elsewhere with two healthy children, didn't I? My mind seemed to resist the knowledge that, yet again, Florence had convulsed. Probably because I didn't want to face what I knew that knowledge meant – that the road to health for Florence still had some way to go; and that the journey that lay ahead of us was through unknown and perilous lands. No one could tell me what was going to happen next.

Seeing my tense face with the eyes threateningly full of the ever-present tears, one of the crew tried to reassure me. Don't worry, lots of children have febrile convulsions, she told me, smiling. I know, I replied. This is Florence's fifth. Oh, she replied. In that case, it's probably something else. They'll probably investigate her for epilepsy.

My heart turned over. Not only had we not made our goal of six convulsion-free months, we were now embarking on a new leg of the journey: that of medical staff acknowledging that the convulsions Florence was having were not straightforward febrile convulsions, but something more. I had known that for a while, but it was a new turn to hear it from them. In the heart of Florence's first illness in May, I'd longed for someone to tell me they weren't just febrile convulsions, would have fallen at their feet and hailed them as some divine overlord if they had decided not to fob me off with the same 'don't know' diagnosis. Now, someone was, but I had judged how I would react quite wrongly. Instead of feeling relieved that we might be on the right path towards diagnosing Florence, I felt terrified for her future.

Not wanting to convey this to Florence, I shut down my thoughts and concentrated on the moment. The ambulance was pulling into the hospital. I cuddled Florence closer. I no longer automatically assumed the hospital was the place to help us, yet I didn't have the confidence to see Florence through a fit and keep her at home without a professional diagnosis. I was living in the no-man's land of waning confidence in the medical profession, but with no real alternative to replace them. I felt I had no choice but to go. Although Johnny had questioned whether we needed an ambulance, I had felt we couldn't risk going it alone. What if we kept her at home and she suffered brain damage? What if my instinct was completely wrong, and it was nothing to do with the vaccine, but meningitis instead, that notorious causer of convulsions and rapid stealer of children's lives? I couldn't take the responsibility. I had no option but to take a walk amongst the white coats.

Once in Casualty, little had changed in five months. Hundreds of battles for lives had been fought here, some won, some lost, since we had last visited, on the day when a man had bled to death before our eyes and a crack cocaine addict had – what, recovered sufficiently to risk another dose? Expired? Who knew, but that was the company we were keeping. We were in Death's Dark Valley, lost in the Jurassic Park of the hospital world without a map and Raptors at every turn.

Ushered along a corridor towards a familiar-looking but different dismal little cubicle, I could see through the glass panels in two swing doors into the shiny new Paediatric Casualty. I remembered my stepmother Marie campaigning to raise money for the unit, her love for her grandchildren igniting her awareness to its need. I remember making a donation. Now, thanks to huge fundraising efforts, it was a reality, a casualty unit designed just for children, to minimise the very real emotional trauma small patients suffered from seeing the harsh aspects of real life on full display in Grown Up Casualty. Through the doors I could see a spotless play area full of new toys, and colourful little cubicles with televisions.

Depressingly, it was closed. I asked the nurse why. She told me there wasn't sufficient money to staff it through the night. Opening hours were 9am until 5pm. Daytime hours, almost identical to a doctor's surgery, the hours when a mother with a sick child might have a chance of getting in to see her GP. 'What about the midnight hours?' I wanted to shout. Didn't doctors know that children always seemed to get seriously sick at night? Didn't Tony Blair have a few kids of his own, or was he so busy being a politician he wasn't aware of their state of health? I couldn't be the only mother who had been forced to turn to Casualty in the early hours. From personal experience, I knew several friends with small children who had, like me, sat anxiously on a trolley bed in the early hours, pleating the sheets nervously between their fingers while cuddled up with their sick child trying to wait patiently for their turn.

But it's hard to wait patiently at Casualty when it's your child that is sick. We'd been there for over an hour – nothing in Casualty terms – and Florence was listless, coughing, and hot. I dreaded another convulsion. There was nothing left to take off her, she was only wearing a pair of cotton pants. But she could have some more Calpol. I considered whether to give it to her myself, or whether to mention it to the nurse who had admitted us. I poked my head out of the cubicle as a rather grey-looking junior doctor of about 25 was about to come in. He smiled at me in a way that had no impact on dispersing the cloak of exhaustion that was almost visibly draped over him.

'Hello,' he said.

I told him our story. His eyes blinked rapidly as he tried to absorb and retain the detail.

He agreed with me that she should have some Calpol. He looked at the bottle, reading the label for dose instructions. I hadn't been to medical school, but the six-hourly dose for Florence was indelibly lodged in my consciousness.

Some more rapid blinking. 'I'm sorry,' he said finally. 'I'm so tired I'm having trouble calculating ...'

'Seven and a half mls.' I said helpfully. 'She can have seven and a half mls.'

He nodded gratefully.

'I'll just check with my colleague.' He called a nurse over. She agreed with me.

We gave Florence seven and a half mls.

The doctor mumbled about arranging our transfer to Paediatric Casualty when it opened at nine. I thanked him, and sat back on the bed with Florence. I now saw with chilling clarity how critical mistakes were made at hospitals. I might think I was tired after a restless, worry-filled night with Florence, but this doctor, he was clearly exhausted. His shift, however long it was, was clearly too long.

At 9am, when Paediatric Casualty finally opened, we walked the few yards along the corridor into this primary-coloured child-oriented world. I collapsed onto a tiny chair intended for a bottom 30 years younger and considerably smaller than mine, in the toy area full of colourful foam building blocks. Florence just looked at them, thumb in mouth.

Soon, a young paediatrician, thankfully refreshingly alert, so presumably at the start of his shift, took down our details once more. He listened to Florence's chest and told me he thought she had pneumonia, although he wanted an X-ray done to confirm this. We went through the X-ray room, and Flo lay down, a pitifully small figure on the large X-ray table, while I stood with her in a lead jacket protecting me from the danger of the rays aimed at my daughter.

The X-ray told the doctor what he wanted to know. Yes, he said, she definitely had pneumonia, he could see the crackles in the lungs. He gave us antibiotics, and said that although he'd ideally like to keep us in, he'd rung up to the children's ward and there just weren't any beds. Could I manage at home? he asked. The question was clearly rhetorical.

I both dreaded and longed to return home. Home was what I knew, and an environment I could control. But frustratingly, however hard I tried I couldn't control Florence's health; for that I needed the back-up of a hospital. I said that I hoped she wouldn't have another convulsion. The doctor shrugged his shoulders. He didn't have a crystal ball, and with her past history, it was possible.

I mentioned then what the ambulance lady had said to me about epilepsy. He nodded in agreement. He told me that the number of fits Florence had had did make it very unlikely that these were simple febrile convulsions. Investigating her for epilepsy was a good idea, but did I have private health care, because the NHS didn't have the resources to do this for us at Florence's stage. I wondered aloud how many potentially brain-damaging fits Florence would have to have before the NHS considered her worth the financial investment. He smiled at me understandingly. We were fleetingly on the same side, lamenting the steady decline of our country's public health system.

Once home, Florence slept on my bed, waking at midday and declaring herself to be hungry. I'd made some chicken noodle soup, the only Jewish dish – in fact very possibly the only dish of any kind – I'd learned to cook well during my marriage to Johnny. This saved his mother dropping a vat of what she termed Jewish Penicillin round every time one of us was ill. Flo came down to the kitchen and we sat together while she sipped at her soup. After three sips she slid off her chair and started to cross the room to the fridge. 'What do you want, darling? Mummy can get it,' I said. But she didn't answer. Mid-stride, her body crumpled like a child shot at play in a war zone. Once on the floor it was clear she was convulsing violently. In horror I scooped her up and carried her through to the sitting room, laying her gently on the sofa.

As Florence lay there twitching and jerking, I wondered how often I was going to see this devastating sight. Were the fits going to become more and more frequent, as the man from JABS had predicted they might? Was Florence's future going to be one of continued and prolonged uncertainty, a slowly unfolding tale of deteriorating health?

I had, like most mothers, unconsciously mapped out a few key images in my head for Florence as she grew up – her first day at school, Florence having her bat mitzvah, Florence growing towards adulthood, possibly even Florence getting married. I had imagined our adult daughter–mother relationship, with us meeting for lunch occasionally or going shopping together, and, eventually, being the grandmother to her children. Now, watching her limbs jerking and teeth grinding, I dreaded that none of these landmarks would be passed. I gave in to the weight of my despair. Tears rolled down my cheeks. For the first time during a convulsion, I allowed myself to cry. After all, what did it matter if I wasn't brave? Florence, unconscious on the sofa, couldn't see my weakness. The tears fell, splashing onto Flo's naked torso.

Meanwhile, Rosalina, our twice-weekly housekeeper, had managed to ring Johnny. Within minutes he was home, anger an inadequate veil over his fear. He stamped about the sitting room, cursing the doctor who had sent me home, wondering aloud why we had to always manage this alone. Agreeing with him, feeling desperate for some medical back-up and reassurance, I asked Johnny to ring our private GP. The GP said he would arrange for our admission to a private London hospital, and that we should go there straightaway.

Strengthened by a plan of action, I wrapped a by now conscious, crying and confused Florence in her dressing gown and climbed with her into the back of the car. I had always insisted my children sat in their car seats. Now I was unable to let Florence go. Johnny, bewildered and frightened, drove his anxious little cargo to the hospital just minutes away.

The hospital admitted Florence quickly, and Johnny and I began to breathe a little easier, reassured by the bottles of oxygen standing by. The inability of the nurse to speak English, however, was a blow. Miming out our concerns seemed to give the whole crisis a ludicrous edge. Was this just another step on our learning curve that hospitals weren't necessarily places to make a person better? Our experiences with the NHS had been so mixed, with top-notch ambulance crews, charming hospital staff literally dropping from exhaustion, and consultants who repeatedly sent us home, for us only to watch Florence fit again.

Once, not so long ago, we'd felt confident that a hospital was the place to make Florence better. Now, even at a private hospital, which had a bed for us only because we were paying, I didn't feel sure that this nurse, with whom I couldn't communicate, would be able to help Florence if the worst happened. Would the instructions on the oxygen bottle be in English? Would she know what to do with it? Would she even understand the word 'Help'?

Flattened with worry about Florence, Johnny and I decided we had no choice but to dismiss these fears and hope the service was going to be more competent than at first glance. At least we were in a medical place. And our paediatrician Ian Hay, who we liked and trusted, was going to visit us here. We just had to hang on.

Florence fell asleep on her bed. Ian Hay arrived. Relieved to see him, I gave him the latest details. We discussed our options. Were these really febrile convulsions Florence was having? Children usually only had one, or two at most, before outgrowing them. The length of some of Florence's convulsions, plus the number, together with the fact that she'd twice had what Ian termed multiple convulsions in one episode – one illness provoking more than one convulsion – suggested there might be another more suitable diagnosis out there. I sensed we were moving towards that umbrella term 'Epilepsy'.

Ian recommended that Florence have a scan to monitor her brain activity, and that we also make contact with a paediatric neurologist for their opinion on the results. We took his advice, and were given an appointment for the following week at Great Ormond Street Hospital. The hospital where really sick children go. The closest any mother wants to come to this hospital is the dropping of a pound coin into a Great Ormond Street collection box.

PEOPLE OPERATE DIFFERENT emotional coping strategies. Some are bottlers, keeping everything to themselves, smiling outwardly, standing firm. Others talk incessantly about what they are going through. The first type are the ones who are war heroes in movies or the brave heroine in a love story. I always wanted to be that type. The leader type, the type to look up to, the best foot forward, Pollyanna type. But I had discovered by now through Florence's illness that I was cast in the second mould. I was the talker, the spill-your-guts type.

Humiliating to have to abandon all those dreams of saving the world in a crisis, but no point going against the flow. Once home the next day, I rang my really close girlfriends one by one and talked the whole nightmare through. Like the friends they truly were and are, they listened patiently and never once indicated boredom or articulated a list of several things they'd rather be doing, like cleaning hair out of the bathroom plug or plucking their eyebrows extremely painfully. On I went in a blow-by-blow account of the latest developments in the ongoing Florence saga. I told them of my fears for her future, my burgeoning doubts in conventional medicine, my lack of anywhere else to turn. What about alternative medicine? Was it voodoo, or could there be something there to help Florence?

Two of them gave me advice that became key in my struggle to help Florence.

My oldest friend Clare told me about a friend of hers whose little boy had developed leukaemia. This mother had just kept on looking for someone to help her, believing the right person was out there somewhere with a cure. That little boy is now a healthy teenager. The message I extracted from this conversation was, keep looking, keep talking, rule nothing out. I just had to keep going.

So far, I had taken Florence down the conventional medicine route, with the exception of her regularly seeing my cranial osteopath Michael Skipwith, whom she had known since birth. The time had surely come to explore the other kinds of help the alternative medicine world had to offer. It was time to open up my probably rather blinkered eyes to homeopathy, Reiki, even hands-on healing. I decided to suspend cynicism, after all I was more than ready for a miracle. Where was the harm in trying? It would cost me time and money, but what I had of those were, needless to say, at my daughter's disposal. I resolved to look into this the very next morning, but where to start?

The answer to this question came the same evening from Gabs, another girlfriend, who was brought up by a mother with a passionate belief in homeopathy and had never had an injection or a course of antibiotics during her childhood.

'Choose the person you trust most in all of this and let them guide you,' she said. 'You need a sense of direction.'

I felt the answer unfurl in my mind: it had to be Michael Skipwith. He knew Florence and he knew her story from me, spilled during our regular appointments. He had treated her as best he could, balancing her system and making suggestions to me that might improve her health. These included taking echinacea, steering clear of dairy products, and giving her lots of rest. He was very well connected in the alternative medicine world, and the obvious person to turn to for advice. Who better to consult about a referral?

I went upstairs to my study to collect my e-mails. News travels fast, and I had lots of e-mails from friends and family concerned about Florence. Several of them shared a common thread: the senders were praying for Florence. My sister Rosie was praying for her recovery, as was my old schoolfriend Briane. Other friends and family were mentioning Florence in their prayers. As I read the messages, I started to cry, not from sheer panic and fear this time, as I had the day before. This weeping was more cathartic, calmer, almost healing, and just a response to so much love, to the support being offered by my family and friends. Most of the time we operate in a world where we think people are too busy to care, to be interested. From my experience with Florence, I now know that isn't so.

My previously held, hazily assembled ideas of life were being overturned one by one in a single evening. Religion had certainly never played much of a part in my life. I was christened as a baby, but actively chose not to get confirmed as a teenager when given the choice at boarding school. I had married a Jewish man in a secular ceremony, and allowed my husband to raise our children as Jews, feeling if there was a God, it was the same God and so he would surely not mind.

And yet here were my friends and family, most of whom seemed about as unreligious as myself, praying for my child in their own ways. The knowledge made me smile through my tears, for hadn't I been praying silently for Florence through every crisis? How many thoughts had started, Please God, give me my daughter back? I had lost count. I only knew that I wouldn't pronounce again in my loud and bossy way that I didn't believe in God. I would be more thoughtful in future, I resolved. My beliefs might not tally with an orthodox organised religious point of view, but I knew now in my heart that He was out there, and that He was listening. In a secular world, when I really hadn't given Him much thought for more than three decades, He was nevertheless still thinking of me.

When I explained this to Johnny, I suspect he thought I'd finally tipped over the edge, had consciously stepped across the fine line that distinguishes the mentally well from the mentally unbalanced. Not wanting to disturb me further, he made some innocuous remark and changed the subject. I remember laughing, knowing exactly what he was thinking. How could I blame him? It was a cliché that people found a higher belief at a time of stress. A comfort when nothing else could help them.

All the same, I went to bed that night drawing comfort from the knowledge that I had changed in a small but profound way.

IT WAS ABOUT this time I had a conversation with my mother that set my mind thinking in a new direction. She had rung up to find out how Florence was, and to tell me that she didn't know if she'd mentioned it before, but was I aware that, 20-odd years ago, one of my sisters, with strawberry blonde hair, had reacted badly to a vaccine?

Something clunked in the pit of my stomach. Florence had had strawberry blonde hair. Could it be that we had a family predisposition to vaccine reaction? Could such a thing be possible? Thinking logically, people did react to medication differently on a person-by-person basis. For example, one glass of wine for one person equalled the effect of two in another. Some people could eat nuts till the cows came home, while others went into life-threatening shock at the mere whiff of a peanut. People did have allergies to different things, and allergies tended to run in families. What if our family was wired in such a way that some of us couldn't cope with vaccination? I thought quickly of my brother, with Crohn's disease, and my father with asthma. I myself have eczema. Put that together with a history of febrile convulsions, and wasn't there just the germ of a theory there?

FLORENCE AND I had got used to being together most of the day, just her and me by now. Occasionally in the last few months I had briefly flirted with the idea of finding some childcare and taking up some part-time work from home again. This, I reasoned, would make me more balanced, giving me a reaffirmed sense of self, and some time thinking about something other than Florence's health.

A flurry of phone calls to nanny agencies would follow, and soon the CVs of Australian girls on gap years, and Sloanes with cooking courses and nanny certificates to their credit but no home of their own to put them to good use in, would start burbling out of the fax machine. Johnny, ever supportive, would help me go through them. We'd select a few to interview.

These interviews were never successful. The candidates never wanted our job. The agency would always try and fudge it – 'She liked you very much, but another job came along that just seemed more right for her' – but Johnny and I both knew what had happened. I had terrified her. Scared her off with tales of Florence's convulsions, followed by a tour of the house revealing doses of her diazepam suppository secreted in various nooks and crannies on all the floors, like a drug addict's secret stash. No sane girl on a gap year would want to take on me, let alone Flo.

She probably thought I was a mad, over-anxious mother. I secretly considered myself to be a mad, over-anxious mother. But with no candidates queuing up to take our job, reassured that no one could look after Florence except myself, the nanny hunt would be called off and life would resume as normal.

So it was just Florence and I who set off in a minicab to Great Ormond Street the following week for her EEG scan. I registered at reception and we went on some long meander involving several corridors and two lifts before arriving at the EEG department. Florence sat on my lap while electrode pads were attached to her head with a gel, with wires leading from them connecting to a machine. These then produced a pattern of her brain activity for a computer to decipher. She looked like something from an alien movie, but complied meekly, sitting on my lap for the duration of the test sucking her thumb. After about 40 minutes of studying the waves intensely, the nurse, giving us no clues as to what she had seen, told us we'd get the results within a week. Florence had all the suckers removed from her head, and we went home.

I tried not to think about what those results might tell us, but rang Ian to see if there was any way of getting the results sooner. Then I pretended it was life as normal. Florence and I took our usual walks in the park to visit the overfed greedy birds who lived on the Round Pond and feed them further.

Four days later, I was in a playpark in Hyde Park with Florence, my friend Clare and her son Leo, on a particularly beautiful late autumn day, the kind that England is so good at. Just when you think there's nothing but grey winter ahead for months, the weatherman pulls out an ace and it's all brilliant blue skies and sunlight that you can actually feel warming your face.

I had adopted a new policy of not droning on incessantly about my problems on the basis that it was (a) bad for me to obsess about Florence and (b) very boring for my friends. I was trying instead to maintain an orderly front to my day, as if I was merely the full-time mother of a regular child rather than the full-time mother of one who convulsed lengthily and scarily at the drop of a hat. When my mobile throbbed through my coat pocket, I gave Florence an extra big push on the swing which she was in, and took a few paces back to answer it. It was Ian's secretary on the phone. The result of Florence's EEG showed no signs of epilepsy. Although this didn't mean she wasn't epileptic, the secretary warned, only that there had been no evidence of epileptic activity during the 40 minutes her brain activity had been monitored, it was nevertheless Good News. For the result also showed that as far as the EEG could pick up, Florence had survived the six convulsions to date, whatever their cause, unscathed. There was no sign of scarring on her brain, and if there had been any, this probably would have shown up on the scan.

I thanked Ian's secretary extremely politely several times as, predictably, my eyes began to water. As a child, my parents had nicknamed me 'Taps' because I cried so often. It seemed that this nickname required reviving. I couldn't trust myself to tell Clare straightaway. I knew I would break down completely. I just watched Florence shrieking with laughter in the swing, her face shining in the late autumn sunlight, and thought, thank you, God. Thank you.

On the basis of this result, the second paediatric neurologist we saw recommended that we should still treat Florence's convulsions as febrile, and, as before, keep a very close eye on fevers. With the back-up of her EEG test, we felt more confident than we had since the whole nightmare had begun back in May.

I also drew comfort from having another angle to explore. I had not forgotten my decision to take a look at what alternative medicine had to offer. I had spoken to Michael about this, and he had recommended me to a homeopath, with whom I had made an appointment.

The day came round, and Florence and I set off to his central London address by minicab, a form of transport to which we had become accustomed given the legal parking potential available in most of London (none).

In his sixties, bearded, he had a gentle manner and a big laugh, and seemed to represent in one person all the Father Christmases I'd ever met. He listened to my story with great attention and sympathy, and when I mentioned the meningitis C vaccine, he shook his head and muttered darkly. This was a new experience for me, as aside from Michael, I had yet to meet someone who didn't dismiss out of hand my by now unshakeable point of view that it had been the meningitis C vaccine that had caused all of Florence's problems in the first place. But this man, with his comforting presence and enquiring manner, didn't seem to consider me as mad as a bag of snakes and unable to control temperature to boot, but to think instead that I might just possibly have a valid point.

He also examined Florence and asked me several detailed questions about her, before writing out a prescription. He gave Florence a little bottle of white pills labelled Thuja, which he told me was the classical remedy given to neutralise the side effects of immunisation. Originally, he said, Thuja had been used to discharge the side effects of vaccination – vaccination meaning smallpox in this case, as that was the origin of the word.

He told me how to give the pills to her – by tipping them into the lid of the bottle and from there into Florence's mouth, as handling reduced their potency. He also warned me not to give Florence chocolate or anything menthol as this interfered with the efficacy of the treatment, and reassured me that there would be no side effects. (I didn't need any more of those.) But homeopathy, he explained, didn't have side effects, and most of the time homeopathic treatment could be run concurrently with conventional treatment.

I gathered up my bag and umbrella from the waiting room, and Florence and I descended slowly in the old-fashioned lift. Outside, we hailed a taxi, and got in to return home. Sitting back in the dark leather seat, with a quiet thumb-sucking Florence belted in beside me, I spent a moment trying to identify the strange, familiar yet unfamiliar feeling that was flapping in my chest like a trapped bird. After a moment, I realised with astonishment that it was hope.

In the past rollercoaster few months, I had felt flooded with relief on a variety of occasions, given into panic on a couple, and fought it off more than that, but this was the first time hope had paid me a visit for quite a while. Hope that one day we might all get through this, and live a normal family life again. I felt like Noah spotting the white dove with an olive branch after months of lashing rain.

SOME PEOPLE ARE really good planners. They do things like book their next Christmas holiday when the one they are enjoying is merely drawing to a close. Johnny and I are many things to each other, and complement each other in a balance of strengths and weaknesses in several areas, but when it comes to planning, we both fall down. We usually book a holiday two weeks before we take it, and it's not unknown for my father to say 'Let me know what you're doing when you've done it', on the basis that that's the earliest I'll have a concrete idea of what our plans might be.

So it was inexplicable to us that we found ourselves in the situation of having uncharacteristically booked a holiday to Mauritius for Christmas months before the Florence problem began. It was a huge step out of character, but somehow, we were committed. We were going with a party of friends, and if we were going to let them down, we had to say so now.

Johnny was extremely keen. A close friend of his was involved in the hotel, and we'd been offered a special reduction in rates because it was apparently running behind schedule and only half built. I had visions of diggers starting work at 6am. Johnny painted pictures of sun and fresh air, and flagged up the positive health benefits for all of us, but most especially Florence.

One of the problems was me. I was frightened of going so far away from our support network – after all, Bath had been too far and that had been just 100 miles away – a network that was at last seeming quite established in the way we needed it to be. I now had a 24-hour GP, a dedicated paediatrician, an osteopath, a homeopath … very Edina from *Absolutely Fabulous*, but I could take the ribbing if it helped Florence.

I also worried about the flight. It was a night flight, and Mauritius had a four-hour time difference to England. Florence would be jet-lagged and tired, and this in turn would suppress her immune system. Wouldn't I be leaving her more vulnerable to infection and possibly yet another convulsion? And if she had one as a result of a whim to go on a holiday, I'd feel more guilty than I already did every single day for having given her the wretched jab that had caused her illness in the first place.

As Johnny and I discussed the pros and cons over a bottle of wine and a take-away curry, we agreed that we'd let Michael and Ian decide. I'd ring them the next day, and see what they recommended.

Both said we should go. I allowed myself to get a little excited. In just a few days, we were heading for the sun. But first, we had a round of events to get through, a series of hurdles that sound like fun when some well-meaning friend suggests them in September, but come the day seem to be just one more thing to accomplish on the stagger to the finishing line that is the end of the year. All this is of course intensified with a child of questionable health in tow.

One such event stands out in my mind as typifying how much we were living on our nerves by then. Johnny's brother and his wife had invited the four of us to Harrods for a special Christmas breakfast the Sunday before Christmas. Their two elder children are of similar age to Jacob and Florence, and it had seemed a nice idea at the time.

Unfortunately, the day dawned on a listless, under-slept Florence, which meant in turn that my waking thought was to question the wisdom of the proposed outing. But Johnny, who possibly saw it as his role to sustain as much normality as possible during those difficult months, insisted that Florence was just tired and that we should honour our social obligation and go.

So we did, and I regretted it from the outset of the taxi ride there. Florence clung to me tiredly through the taxi ride and the inevitable queue to get in, and sat limply on my knee throughout the breakfast. She cringed away from Father Christmas when he bellowed a well-meaning 'Ho Ho Ho' at close range. I, meanwhile, barely had the digital thermometer out of her ear. I was sure she was hot. After half an hour, my worst fears were confirmed. Her temperature was rising.

'I'm going to find the loo and cool her down with some water,' I said, wishing like mad I was at home.

I rushed off with Florence in my arms, away from the restaurant and through the toy department, beyond which I knew were the loos.

Very soon I found myself in the eerie gloom of a closed toy department. I could wander through, but the store lights were out. It was clear that while Harrods was open for breakfast, it certainly wasn't open for shopping. There wasn't a person in sight. I pushed on to the loos, only to find them locked. I couldn't stand it. Staggering under Flo's weight, I fantasised about putting her in a cool bath at home. Why had I let myself be persuaded to take her out? Yet another bad decision, I berated myself.

'Help me someone,' I yelled, utterly lost now, surrounded by a rather spooky-looking family of larger-than-life stuffed bears.

'Darling, I'm here,' called Johnny, dashing into the room. 'I've been looking for you everywhere.'

He took Flo from me and together we headed to the lift. Johnny had arranged for Jacob to stay with his brother while he found Flo and me and put us in a cab.

'I could come with you,' he offered.

'No, you make sure Jacob has a good time,' I replied. 'Keep your phone on and I'll call you.'

Florence and I made it home and into that much-fantasised about lukewarm bath. Her temperature came down. When Johnny and Jacob came home two hours later, they found us curled up on the rug watching *Mary Poppins*.

But as an episode it serves as an example of how all family life was truncated by both the fear and the reality of Florence's illness.

Johnny and I, amazingly, barely fought about our management of it. But Jacob undoubtedly missed out on the calm of a family home where one child is not permanently at least semi-sick. That year, he missed a lot of the mundane little episodes that make up a child's rock-steady life, instead his mother riding off at no notice whatsoever in ambulances with his sister cradled in her arms. Too often that year I found myself saying 'Not now, Jakey, I've just got to look after Flo' as I panicked yet again about a slight rising temperature and what it could mean for her.

THE WEEK BEFORE Christmas we shrugged off the London damp like an old mac and flew out to Mauritius. The hotel turned out to be exquisite. Our two connecting rooms overlooked the sea and had a little private terrace. There was a spa, two fabulous pools and several tennis courts. The food was delicious, and in our party of 20 were several other children for Jacob and Florence to play with. Because only some of the rooms were ready and occupied, the hotel felt really spacious. The staff were really friendly and gently shepherded Jacob back to us when his curiosity led him astray.

Days passed easily. Jacob learned to swim without armbands and was rarely sighted out of the pool. Daily, Florence and I walked the beach filling her pink bucket with shells. Then she made a friend, a little girl a year older than her. This was her first real girlfriend outside family, and the sight of her little swimsuit-clad figure earnestly talking Barbies for hours on end with Hannah made me blush with pleasure. Was it possible that after all she'd been through she was, after all, going to have a normal childhood, leading to a full and busy life? Somehow I hadn't noticed until recently that her hair had started to grow back, although it was blonde and curly this time, as opposed to her previous strawberry blonde and straight.

But that must be a sign of health, I thought. And she was eating well and her energy levels seemed to be increasing daily.

On the last day of the holiday, a few days after we'd waved Hannah goodbye, Florence told me that she wanted to go back to nursery school. 'Like Hannah, Mummy' she told me. I knew then, as I had in September, that I shouldn't allow my fears to hold her back. I had to allow her to grow, make friends, develop. She needed more than me and my close, protective little world. But then, our attempt had failed. Would it fail again? All those bugs she'd be exposed to at nursery. All those bugs that might lead to serious illness and convulsion. I looked again into her pink, smiling little face. It was no good. I couldn't deny her. Everyone said we had to live as normally as possible – Ian Hay, Michael Skipwith, plus an army of friends and relatives with an opinion. I had to swallow my fear once again and face it.

We flew home, a family seemingly restored to health and vitality, transformed by a three-week break. We tumbled headlong into London life. Just a few days later, Jacob had to be coerced into a stiff new grey shirt and wear a tie for the first time in his life. He was going to Big School, and wasn't remotely keen. Johnny, sensing a Difficult Family Moment, had conveniently absented himself to the Peak District on urgent business for a few days. The job of frog-marching a weeping Jacob to his first day was left to me.

I duly did so, leaving him weeping in his new classroom. The rest of that day, haunted by images of Jacob standing alone in the playground, Jacob crying into his sponge and custard that he wanted to go home, I made enquiries about a suitable small, nursery school for Florence. I didn't want her to go back to the Montessori she'd so briefly started at. Right though it had been for Jacob, it felt too big and impersonal to contain a potential problem like Flo's. I wanted a small, cosy little nursery, that would notice if she was tired or quiet, and ring me.

My mother-in-law told me about a friend of hers who ran a little nursery just five minutes drive away. Johnny and I rang up, and booked to go for a visit.

We took Florence with us. The nursery was small, and Johnny made lots of jokes about bumping into the lampshades (he's six foot four) and feeling like Alice in Wonderland after she's eaten the Grow Big Cake.

We watched the five, smiling teachers and the 20 children at work and at play, while Florence was invited to explore the little play kitchen. The atmosphere was calm, controlled and happy. I talked with the head about Florence's health. She said they could cope with special needs. An autistic boy came twice a week, she told me, and they had once had a boy with cystic fibrosis who had needed oxygen regularly. Listening to her talk, and observing the way the teachers related to the children, I really believed her. It seemed we had found the perfect place for Florence, a safe place for her to develop and grow. Now we just had to hope there was room for her. The head told me she'd know next week. Apparently a child might be leaving to go back to Sweden.

A few days later, during the fast-becoming-normal wrestling match that was laughingly known as 'getting Jacob ready for school', Florence complained to me of a headache. Johnny left to take the reluctant Jacob to school, while Florence settled on the sofa to watch the Tweenies. She asked me for some bagel with honey on. As I turned towards the kitchen, I heard a whoop noise. I knew what it was, even though I didn't want to acknowledge it. I even went as far as saying to myself, I wonder what that noise is?

All in a split second. For I knew precisely what sort of noise it was. It was the sound a child made when their eyeballs were rolling back in their head and their body starting to convulse. I could hardly bear to face the fact that I was hearing it again. I wanted to turn round and see Florence sitting up on the sofa, smiling at me.

Instead, she was slowly sliding off it, unconscious. I caught her before she hit the floor.

By the time Johnny was back from dropping Jacob at school, Florence was awake and grizzly, confused, aware something had happened to her but not sure what. Johnny threw his hands up on hearing that it had happened yet again. When was this ever going to end? he shouted in despair. I utterly took his point, but pointed out that at least it was a short fit, certainly the shortest by some way since this nightmare had started, and she had recovered quickly.

Inside I was despairing. The gap between the fits was closing, just as the man from JABS had warned they might. This one was just ten weeks after the last. Were we, as I'd dreaded in my darkest, most alone moments, on the downhill slide?

The phone rang. Johnny answered it furiously. 'YES?!' he bellowed at the unsuspecting caller. With the timing that only Life can perfect, it was The Gate nursery, offering Florence a place to start after half-term.

Chapter Seven

Andrew Wakefield and the MMR

The MMR is the triple vaccine, given to children to protect them against measles, mumps and rubella, that has been at the top of the list of parents' vaccination concerns for some years. Ever since early 1998, when Andrew Wakefield, a British gastroenterologist at the Royal Free Hospital in London, went public with his theory that there might be a link between the MMR and a new kind of regressive autism with bowel disease, confusion over this jab has reigned – and not just amongst parents: the medical and scientific professions are divided over the safety profile of the jab.

Wakefield's scientific sample, on which he based his original supposition, was small – just 12 children – and he was the first to admit that such a link was only a possibility, not a fact. But these 12 children, aged between three and ten, all had had a history of normal development, followed by a regression that included the loss of skills including language, and accompanied by bowel problems. Parents of eight of these children told Wakefield that their child's deterioration in health had followed the MMR.

Making it quite clear that he was not anti-vaccination, and had no interest in leaving children unprotected against measles, Wakefield called for more research to be done to establish whether his doubts about the MMR were grounded. In the meantime, until research concluded one way or the other, he recommended that children should have single vaccines.

Such a statement was never going to be popular – either with the drug companies who supply the MMR (and the majority of funding for scientific research) or with the Department of Health, who have consistently promoted the safety and effectiveness of the MMR – and it would prove to be a turning point for Wakefield's career in the UK.

Wakefield worked on, identifying more children with similar symptoms of autism and bowel disorders to the original 12 he had examined. By the year 2000, Wakefield had studied 150 children with what he termed 'autistic enterocolitis' – a new type of regressive autism accompanied by bowel disease. He had also found that biopsies from the guts of a group of 25 children displaying such symptoms showed that 24 of them had the live measles virus in their gut.

Following injection with a live virus vaccine like measles, a child's immune system should mount a defence to the virus, and destroy the virus cells within a few weeks. But in these children, for some reason, this was not happening. Instead, the virus was remaining live within them. Was it the presence of this virus in their bodies that was causing the degeneration in their health? None of these children had ever had wild measles. Their only exposure to measles had been through the MMR, which meant that almost certainly the virus had entered their bodies through an injection.

Theories began to circulate. Was it the giving of three live viruses at once that was the problem? Did this overwhelm the immune systems of some children, allowing the measles virus to persist in their bodies? After all, the measles virus was known to suppress the immune system temporarily.

The Department of Health sought to reassure the public on this issue: the MMR was quite safe; a child's body could cope with many germs at one time, they said. Meanwhile, as word of Wakefield's research spread, more children were being referred to the Royal Free with similar sets of symptoms.

But Wakefield's work, so challenging to the credibility of the MMR, was increasingly controversial. Finally, Wakefield left the Royal Free Hospital and went to America to continue his work. The Royal Free has since put a stop to the research it was doing into the link between the MMR and the new kind of autism with bowel disease.

Nevertheless, the uncertainty surrounding the MMR has remained.

Parents versus the MMR manufacturers

Wakefield's 1998 paper may have fully ignited the public debate on the MMR, a debate that has continued without any signs of resolution since that date, but the truth is that there had been rumbles of concern about the MMR for some years prior to this. Parents had been reporting problems with the triple jab as early as the beginning of the 1990s. A legal case has been gathering steam for some time, brought against the companies who manufacture the MMR, by 1000 parents, some of whom claim that their children were damaged by the MMR as long ago as 1992.

Richard Barr, a medical negligence solicitor, was first approached in 1990, by a mother with the story of her son who had developed meningitis shortly after having his MMR.

In 1992, when the Department of Health withdrew two of the three brands of MMR that were then in use, amid fears that the mumps component caused mild meningitis, several more parents contacted Barr with tales of damage done to their children, they believed, by the vaccine.

In 1994, the government announced that an epidemic of measles was forecast, and that children between five and 16 should receive the measles/rubella vaccine. The two brands used in this mass vaccination programme were produced by the same manufacturers as the two brands of the MMR vaccine that had been withdrawn in 1992. The theory put forward by the medical negligence lawyers is that these measles/rubella vaccines were just the remaining two parts of the withdrawn triple jab. Only the mumps component was missing. The implication here is, were these components, taken from a jab previously withdrawn on safety grounds, up to scratch?

The result is that there are two groups of claimants in the legal case, which is being brought against GlaxoSmithKline, Aventis Pasteur MSD and Merck and Co. – those children who received the MMR vaccine; and those children who received the MR vaccine. The side effects reported include autism, bowel problems, epilepsy, brain damage, menigitis, cerebral palsy, encephalopathy, encephalitis, deafness in one or both ears, multiple sclerosis and behavioural and learning difficulties in older children.

The pharmaceutical companies have mounted a strong defence, including trying –unsuccessfully – to get the case thrown out on technical legal grounds which would, if it had been successful, have prevented the facts being established.

It is a challenging road ahead for Barr and his band of parents. It is hard to impossible to prove that damage to a child is the result of a vaccine, as Richard Barr, heading the team of solicitors, well knows.

'No vaccine claim in this country has yet succeeded. We hope to be the first,' Barr said. As he pointed out: 'These families have to cope with children who were normal before vaccination, but many of whom will never be able to live independently. They will never leave home. They will outlive their parents and many have such serious behaviour problems that they will have to live in institutions after their parents' death.'

The MMR abroad

Britain isn't the only country to have issues with the MMR.

Canada withdrew a version of the MMR in 1990, identical to one withdrawn in Britain in 1992. This was withdrawn amidst fears of a link between the mumps component and meningitis, as Britain acted similarly two years later. Canada uses a different version of MMR today.

Japan has already had its own MMR confidence crisis. Japan withdrew the version of the MMR they were using in 1993, following reports of severe neurological problems. Some 1000 people suffered side effects from MMR, mostly meningitis, and three died. The mumps component of the jab was the source of the problem, and this was a different mumps component to that used in the UK. The Japanese now use single vaccines instead. There has been a rise in measles deaths, but these are apparently largely in children under the age of one, who are too young to have a measles vaccination.

But ten years on, Japan has not reintroduced the MMR. As Channel 4 News journalist Ian Williams reported in 2001: 'Not only has Japan abandoned MMR in favour of the single measles shot, but this has had a wider impact. Such is public disillusion with what's seen as dishonest, bungling bureaucrats that it has undermined public confidence in vaccination.'

Meanwhile, in the United States, the national vaccine compensation programme has paid out over $1 billion in the last ten years in vaccine damage claims, 14 per cent of which has been paid out for MMR or its components. The MMR has clearly provoked some claims of damage over there too.

Conflicting points of view

It is against this historical background that the British battle over the safety or otherwise of the MMR continues. It is a fight that is frequently played out in the national press, meaning parents are widely exposed to a range of MMR stories. It's obviously a valid and important debate, but in the face of so much conflicting opinion many parents don't know what to think when it comes to the MMR.

On the one hand, there are those who support the MMR. This camp includes the World Health Organization, and many respected scientists and experts from around the world, who have variously gone on record stating that they believe there is no link between MMR and autism.

Then there's the UK government. They have remained adamant throughout the controversy that the MMR has no link with autism. The Department of Health literature on the MMR says: 'Extensive research ... shows that there is no link between MMR and autism. These research studies have been carried out in this country, the USA, Sweden and Finland, and involve thousands of children.' The DoH literature also says: 'The MMR was thoroughly tested before it was introduced. There was more than a decade of experience in the US before it was used in the UK.'

This message and many similar ones in support of the MMR, have been widely distributed to the public over the last few years via several heavy marketing campaigns incorporating booklets, videos, leaflets, advertisements and helplines.

But all this has failed to convince the scientists, doctors, professionals and parents who doubt the MMR.

First, the MMR critics have raised one essential question: Is the real, necessary research into any link between autism and the MMR actually being done? In other words, is the government actually looking in the right places for a link between MMR and autism?

One American scientist, Professor Vijendra Singh at Utah State University, who found that autism might be an immune system response to the MMR, made the following criticism of the UK's Public Health Laboratory Service, one of the government's health bodies: 'If they [the PHLS] enter their same old data ... they will continue to find the same old answer, i.e., there is no possibility of a connection between MMR and autistic regression.'

Next, many of the very studies and trials the government cites in defence of the MMR's safety record have also been criticised, sometimes on grounds of bias if they were funded by pharmaceutical companies, sometimes on grounds of quality.

Andrew Wakefield is one person who has claimed that safety trials of the MMR were inadequate. In January 2001, he published a study in *The Lancet*, 'Through a glass darkly', which suggested that the MMR had been introduced without adequate safety trials. He criticised the fact that the vaccine trials only monitored children for three or four weeks, so any side effects which presented after this time would not have been picked up.

Two individuals who had been involved in originally passing the MMR for use back in the late 1980s reviewed this article, and expressed similar concerns themselves. One of these was Dr Peter Fletcher, a former principal medical officer in the Medicines Division, now the Medical Control Agency (MCA), of the Department of Health, who served as a medical assessor to the Committee on the Safety of Medicines (CSM). Writing in *The Lancet*, he said:

> With all the benefits of hindsight, what may now be said about the decision to grant a Product Licence to MMR 10 or so years ago? Evidence on quality and efficacy was probably adequate so a decision had to be made on grounds of safety ... Being extremely generous, evidence on safety was very thin. Being realistic, there were too few patients followed up for insufficient time. Three weeks is not enough ...

Dr Fletcher also commented on the combining of the three viruses: 'There was insufficient information on the immunological effects of a trivalent vaccine compared to monovalent vaccines.'

The second reviewer, Professor Duncan Vere, a former member of the Committee on the Safety of Medicines, was quoted in the *Private Eye* special investigation into the MMR in response to Wakefield's 'Through a glass darkly' article. He said: 'In almost every case, observation periods were too short to include the onset of delayed neurological or other adverse events.'

So those are just some of the views of scientists opposed to the MMR. Then there are the non-scientists who fervently believe the MMR is causing problems for some children.

One such is Paul Shattock, who runs the Autism Research Unit at the University of Sunderland. He told me in an interview:

> There is not just one cause of autism, there are many. But the MMR is one that the finger has been pointed at, and I think it has got to be investigated. Ten to eleven per cent of children with autism in the UK have parents who swear that it was triggered by the MMR. And I believe them.

> This is a regressive autism. The kids are developing normally in every way, and parents have the video recordings to prove it. The first thing the parents notice is the behavioural regression, which takes an average of 15 days to come out. With the second shot, the children often go down the next day.

The figures Shattock provides make for a grim read. 'Current estimates of autism are about one in every 150 children. If ten per cent of that is triggered by the MMR vaccine, then assuming 100 per cent uptake, that is one in every 1500 children being made autistic by the MMR.'

Some GPs have expressed their concern over the MMR. GP Dr Peter Mansfield, one of the first doctors to offer single jabs, told a newspaper that giving three live viruses was like 'opening Pandora's box without any idea of what will fly out'.

Dr Nicholson, GP and editor of the *Bulletin of Medical Ethics*, when I interviewed him in the summer of 2002, said:

> By ordinary scientific standards, we don't have the evidence to say there is no link between autism and the MMR. So far, in the claims to the MMR's safety, we have only had a review of existing papers. Until we have a prospective study looking for the link between MMR and autism and bowel disease, we won't know.

Justice Awareness and Basic Support (JABS), the organisation that seeks to inform parents about all aspects of vaccines, has maintained for years that the MMR is causing damage to children. JABS runs a register for children with vaccine damage. They say on their website that they have 27 children on their registers with vaccine damage attributed to the single measles vaccine, which was given to children from 1967 to 1988; but they have 1700 children with vaccine damage attributed to the MMR, which covers the period from 1988, when the MMR was introduced, to the present day. The implication of these figures is that the MMR is causing many more problems for children than the single measles jab ever did.

Finally, there are the personal stories that can sow powerful seeds of doubt. One particular example stands out. When UK Prime Minister Tony Blair was asked whether his son Leo had had the MMR jab, he refused to answer, claiming it was an invasion of privacy. Given his usual willingness to be seen as a family man (we can all remember the family holiday photo shoots), this protracted refusal led to speculation that Leo had not had the MMR. Otherwise, the feeling was, he would surely have said so. If not, why not? Did Tony know something that other parents didn't?

Is it any wonder that in a recent poll, only 51 per cent of parents said they felt sure the MMR was safe? Parents simply want to make the best decision for their child, but at the moment, it is utterly unclear what that decision is. How can parents be certain when the scientists and medics can't reach agreement? Is it surprising that MMR uptake levels have fallen, that some parents have sought out expensive single jabs, only to hear them criticised on grounds of quality, or that others, frozen with indecision, simply do nothing?

It is obviously vital that these opposing groups fight their way to an end game. But going on past form, it is reasonable to expect this may take years. Where does this leave parents in the meantime?

The government has always maintained that the MMR is the safest way to protect children from measles, mumps and rubella. But this cannot be the case if parents, confused and in doubt as to its safety, refuse to submit their children to the process. Although (licensed, quality-assured) single jabs may leave children unprotected against measles, mumps and rubella for longer than the MMR, given the stalled nature of the MMR debate, they may also, as Wakefield spotted back in 1998, represent a good, if temporary, alternative. That is something for parents to decide. After all, a fact often obscured in the heat of the MMR debate, is that it is they, together with their children, who are the daily victims in this crisis.

Chapter Eight

Florence IV

Recovery Position

Life felt like a ghastly game of Snakes and Ladders. The Ladders represented Hope and consisted of all the positives that happened to us in between convulsions: Florence making a friend, her hair growing back, having more energy, the possibility of nursery school for her, the protective sandbanks of Time that we were hoarding up, distancing us from her last convulsion. All those things boosted us up the board. The convulsions were the venomous, predatory Snakes against whom we had to pit our wits and prayers, and win. The trouble was, were we winning? Sometimes, like in the aftermath of a convulsion, wondering if Florence would remember the name of her favourite Teletubby, it didn't feel like it. It didn't feel like it at all.

Frustratingly, once again, we'd just slid down a Snake. As always when this happened, I needed to make a plan. Taking action made me feel I was doing something positive to tackle the problem, and therefore could cope with it better.

A plan by now meant medical advice and second opinions. I rang Ian Hay, and he said he thought it was time we saw a different paediatric neurologist. He explained that there were two schools of thought in paediatric neurology on convulsions, and we'd seen one person who represented the 'it will right itself' aspect. He recommended we see someone who would outline possible forms of treatment we could consider. After all, he said, Florence had had seven convulsions in as many months. Even on the basis that she would grow out of them at five, she wasn't yet even three. I did the maths: that could mean another 25 convulsions before reaching the age at which she might technically grow out of them.

Twenty-five fits, I thought. What a terrible future for a little girl who should be enjoying her early years. Twenty-five fits, I thought. That's a lot of potential for brain damage. Far too many fits to contend with. Ian Hay made us an emergency appointment with the paediatric neurologist he recommended.

Sitting in the latest paediatric neurologist's office just a few evenings later, we outlined our experiences with Florence. The neurologist was very sympathetic. She told us that while in the UK the general policy was not to put children like Florence who had multiple convulsions on anticonvulsants, in other countries quite the opposite was standard. She gave the US and France as examples.

The benefit of an anticonvulsant, she told us, was that we wouldn't have to worry all the time that another convulsion was around the corner. Johnny and I looked at each other with growing excitement as she painted an enchanting picture in heavenly colours of Florence, Jacob, Johnny and myself living a normal family life, no longer dogged by the dark threat of a convulsion. No more leaping at shadows, no more doling out the Calpol on a speculative basis. No more family outings-turned-nightmare, like the one before Christmas to Harrods.

Yes! We thought. Why hadn't anyone mentioned this to us before! Well, the paediatric neurologist told us, that's probably because of the side effects.

The balloon of hope collapsed as rapidly as it had inflated. The side effects sounded horrendous. Weight gain, sleepiness, potential liver failure, all more likely in the under-three's. Florence was two years nine months. Could we even consider such an option?

Think it over, the neurologist urged us. And, as a parting shot, she added: 'If it was my child, for what it's worth – I'd risk the side effects.'

We stumbled out into the dark street, a mental image of a swollen dumbed-down Florence sitting listlessly on the sofa for evermore looming much too large in my mind. I told Johnny this, and he confessed he was equally tormented by a Florence brain-damaged from a long untended convulsion. Clichéd talk about being between a rock and a hard place now began to have genuine and heartfelt meaning. Not wanting to parrot Tony Blair, I felt there had to be a Third Way.

The next morning, the hunt for this third alternative began. I visited Michael, and begged him to refer me to someone else he had once mentioned to me, a man called Ravi. Ravi was an iridologist homeopath – that is, he partly diagnosed by looking into the patient's eyes. My sister-in-law had mentioned him to me years before in a rather reverential way after he had helped her with some health problem, and I knew she had found him via Michael.

Michael considered my request for a moment. I wondered why he hadn't sent me to him before. I think I knew the answer already. Because Ravi would see the truth of Florence's condition, and it might be more than I could stand. Michael had already told me he didn't think Florence's fits were straightforward febrile convulsions, but the result of vaccine damage. What he had never hazarded a guess on, to me at least, was where these fits were taking her. Ravi, he left me in no doubt, would shoot from the hip taking no prisoners. 'I'm ready for that,' I said. 'Please, just give me the number.'

I rang the number and spoke to Ravi's unflappable, calm assistant. At first an appointment seemed weeks away, but something in

Florence's story, retold in my steely tones quite possibly tinged with a hysterical edge by now, meant we ended up being given an urgent appointment. We had a week to wait.

In the meantime, trying to cover both fronts of medicine, I also took Florence to see Ian to discuss the anticonvulsants situation. Sharing my fears about the side effects, he agreed we should proceed cautiously. As a preliminary measure, he recommended testing Florence's liver function to see if it was normal. If it wasn't we couldn't consider the anticonvulsants anyway. I agreed to do this right away.

Florence was furious at having the local anaesthetic cream put on her hands and the inside of her elbow and then stuck there with a plaster so she couldn't rub it off. We had to allow the cream 45 minutes to work, and to distract her I took her to a nearby Italian restaurant for a bowl of her favourite pasta and an ice-cream. The Italian waiters fluttered about her, besotted with this small girl child with her little halo of very short golden curls and an Italian's appetite for pasta. While Florence shovelled in her spaghetti and lapped up the attention, I couldn't eat my lunch, unable to take my eyes off her plasters. I felt like I was in a terrible Hollywoodesque tear-jerker, giving my terminally sick child a favourite treat before she died.

An hour later, I tried to concentrate on reading Florence a story as she sat on my lap, with a doctor taking blood from her hand, a process I was trying to conceal from her with the storybook. Florence, despite the cream, knew something horrible was happening to her, and kept twisting her body and craning her neck to see what it was. I was equally determined that she shouldn't catch sight of the needle, the line, or the test tubes rapidly filling with her blood.

It was a pathetic battle that Florence had no hope of winning. I knew that if we put her on sodium valporate, the recommended anticonvulsant that was coincidentally what was used to treat epilepsy, this would become a twice-monthly outing. I felt deeply depressed at the prospect.

That day was a big day for both of us. By coincidence, our appointment with Ravi was that afternoon, so we had to go straight on to Islington afterwards.

Ravi's surgery was in the back of an opticians and looked very unassuming. After a few minutes waiting, a smiling, slim Indian man with lively eyes opened a door and beckoned us into his room. This, apparently, was Ravi. Florence sat on my knee while I explained we had been referred by Michael and that Florence had been having convulsions for just over seven months.

Without further preliminaries he pulled on a pair of what looked like a cross between spectacles and binoculars, and asked to look into Florence's eyes. He quickly began to speak. He told me she had had a bad reaction to a vaccine, and that her liver was loaded with toxins. He said these needed discharging as they were suppressing her immune system, meaning every time she fell even slightly ill the illness quickly became serious and convulsions resulted. He said he could give me something to get rid of the toxins. I was impressed, as I had not yet told him about the meningitis C vaccine being, in my mind, the trigger point for Florence's illness.

When I did, he just nodded, still smiling, very calm, so unworried I wondered whether I could believe his diagnosis. Perhaps he hadn't heard me correctly? Should I tell him again? But my choices were limited at best and what harm could it do anyway? Homeopathy had no side effects. After another ten minutes of conversation about Florence's general health and diet, I told Ravi that we were considering putting her on sodium valporate. His reaction was quiet but clear. Florence was not an epileptic, he told me. However, if I put her on sodium valporate she might become one. There was a chance that once she was on it, I'd never get her off it.

Ravi also told me to stop giving Florence Calpol and Nurofen unless directly responding to a fever. Strangely, this felt like the lifting of a heavy sentence rather than a withdrawal of my only weapon to date against fever. No more would I have to try and dance the right steps with my invisible and rather menacing dancing partner, What If. Instead, I would only treat the actual. I went home clutching a plastic bag full of homeopathic pills and drops, including a homeopathic treatment for fever. I started Florence on them straightaway, and that night Johnny and I sat down to form a plan of action.

I had worried that I'd have to really work to persuade Johnny against the sodium valporate in the light of my afternoon's experience, but it turned out there was no need. He was against it on the basis of the side effects alone. I was relieved. If I'd had to explain that my decision was based on Ravi's opinion, a man whom I'd never met until a few hours ago but was now entrusting with my daughter's health care, I would have struggled. Johnny was deeply cynical about alternative medicine. I think he regarded my visits to Michael and whoever he recommended me to, as something I did to make myself feel better, and on that basis they could be justified, but on no other. A sort of investment in my mental health, was probably how he viewed it, but of absolutely no use to Florence.

That night, we also agreed that we couldn't live from fit to fit like this any more. It was turning our family life into a half-life, a neurotic, permanently on-red-alert life, and it certainly wasn't fair on Jacob.

We decided that if Florence had one more fit, we would move to live by the sea, somewhere like Brighton, at first temporarily, to see if a change of scene would help. It sounded old-fashioned, seeking the sea air-type rest cure, but it also made sense. We both thought that the density of London's germ-carrying population, coupled with the pollution, wasn't the healthiest environment. We planned that if she had another convulsion, I would rent a cottage or apartment with Florence, and Johnny and Jacob would come for the weekends. It comforted us, the knowledge that we had something to do if the unthinkable happened and Florence had yet another convulsion, but both of us hoped we'd never have to do it. We were like citizens in a country preparing for war: we'd been issued gas masks, but were hoping we'd never have to use them.

We also agreed we'd reconsider sodium valporate if the number of Florence's fits reached ten. So far, we were only on seven. That left us with three in hand.

Council-of-war over, we continued with normal life as best we could. Florence seemed to have a little more energy each day, although she probably still spent too long tucking herself up on the sofa claiming to be tired. Johnny and I worried we'd over-coddled her, that she was taking her lead from us. More guilt.

My mother-in-law, meanwhile, in a gesture that let me know she appreciated something of what I was going through, sent me a huge voucher for a top local spa. On receiving it, my body aching with tiredness, tense from continual anxiety, I felt like crying from the sheer kindness of it. It will probably remain one of the best presents I've ever had.

The spa offered evening appointments and I booked in for as soon as possible on nights when Johnny could babysit. At the first appointment, the therapist asked me how I was. 'Oh, fine,' I squeaked conventionally, before finding myself pouring out my tale of woe the very next moment, tears pricking my eyes, of course.

'You certainly need this then,' she said, after listening sympathetically, massaging tension out of my shoulders and somehow miraculously recharging my energy.

I used up the entire voucher within ten days on three fabulously revitalising aromatherapy massages. I'd previously thought massages were just a luxury, a treat you afforded yourself every now and then with no real impact, but those three treatments, three hours of someone else doing things for me, as opposed to my trying to save the world and failing, felt like a refilling of the emotional petrol tank.

I sat on the guilt I felt at taking the time, while Johnny minded Flo. I had to keep going, for all our sakes, so not grasping the opportunity would have been foolish.

Four weeks after our initial visit, I took Florence back to Ravi for a follow-up session. He looked through her eyes again, and said she wasn't absorbing enough calcium and he could give her something for it.

'Yes, yes,' I said, brushing this aside as a secondary issue. (Looking back, I imagine my general tone of voice concerning Florence to have been permanently edged with tension.) 'But what about the convulsions,' I asked. 'She seems to be getting a cold, what can I do to prevent another convulsion?'

'Oh, the convulsions,' Ravi said. 'You don't need to worry about those anymore. She won't have any more convulsions.'

He said it almost casually, as if he were saying 'Oh, don't worry about her in-grown toe nail, it's better now'. Or perhaps that was just my perception, for how could I regard such a statement as anything but critical, life-changing, vital? Convulsions had been ruling our lives for nine months. To say that I didn't need to worry about them, when I'd done nothing but for nearly a year!

I drove all the way home with my mouth open. I turned Ravi's phrase over and over in my mind as I wondered whether I dared to believe it. My brother-in-law said no, another friend said I should. I wanted to, desperately. But like Doubting Thomas, I needed proof. I decided to wait and see. One day at a time.

A month later, after the February half-term, Florence started nursery school. She was so ready for the socialising and the stimulation. The teachers were well-briefed, and calmly confident they could cope if she had a fit. I couldn't bear the idea that she might have a fit when I wasn't there to help her, but equally I knew I had to let her grow a little at a time. I hung on to Ravi's reassurance, and watched as Florence settled quickly. We reached the end of term without incident.

Over Easter, we went to Cornwall. Jacob came down with an ear infection that required antibiotics, and I spent several days on tenterhooks waiting for Florence to get it too, but amazingly she remained well.

Suddenly, we'd notched up three convulsion-free months, and we still had the summer – traditionally a less germy time – ahead of us. We had carefully climbed several Ladders, avoiding the gaping ravenous mouths of the Snakes. It was early days, Johnny and I cautioned each other; but still, she was doing very well.

The summer term began. I was still very cautious, and only sent Florence to school if I was sure she was completely well. Sometimes, I kept her home just because she seemed a little tired. But when she went, she thrived. The teachers were wonderfully supportive. As the weather improved, I began to plan half-term. We'd go to Cornwall, and Florence and I, by way of a little treat, would drive down a day ahead of Jacob and Johnny, who would follow by train.

Florence and I broke our journey in Bath, where I took her to the Victoria Gardens with its huge and exciting play park. We had supper together at seven o'clock in the garden of our hotel, and then we went to sleep together, sharing a big double bed. As I lay in the fading daylight under cool sheets, my daughter's steady breathing lifting then dropping the sheet infinitesimally every few seconds, I felt very blessed. I was doing things that a year ago would have seemed impossible. Normal mother-and-child things, but nevertheless things I had once dreaded would never come to pass. Slowly, quietly, it seemed a future was opening up again for Florence, a future I had dreaded she might not have.

The next day we drove on to Cornwall and spent the afternoon digging in the sand, and paddling in the sea. We ate fish and chips on the harbour wall, before walking back up to the hotel for an early night. I drank a glass of wine on the balcony of our room once Florence was asleep, looking out to sea. It was now five months since her last convulsion, and somehow Florence was making great strides: starting nursery and forming friendships; her hair growing longer, which I took as an indication of her general health; even her increased naughtiness, a trial to most parents, was good news to us. After all, it required energy to be naughty.

While I still worried away, never talking about Florence being well without touching wood, and never managing to talk about her at all for very long without mentioning her illness, the knot of tension within my breast bone that had for months been a part of me, gradually began to ease. Suddenly, the year began to roll ahead smoothly. We had an uneventful summer holiday that at eight weeks was endless but also rushed by like a speeding train, gone in a flash.

By September, I had to admit to myself that Florence seemed a completely normal three-and-a-half-year-old. She could be a delight and a menace, loved dolls and the rough and tumble of play in the house and garden with her brother. She was very determined, and mad keen on having her hair in two plaits. It now hung to her shoulders and she was in competition with Rapunzel. She wanted to grow it down to her bottom.

It took me a further three months really to believe in Florence being well. In the October half-term she had a temperature, but didn't convulse. At Christmas, she had a cough and fought it off. In

January, I took her to see Ravi again. I needed to hear those words once more.

'Ravi,' I began, 'do you remember you said she won't have any more convulsions?' 'She won't have any more convulsions,' he confirmed, smiling at my anxiety but in the nicest possible way.

'Was it really the vaccine that caused it?' I asked.

He nodded. 'You were lucky,' he said. 'I've seen much, much worse.'

Ravi told me he had five healthy children and hasn't vaccinated any of them.

I drove home with those words resounding in my head. I was lucky! I was lucky! We were among the lucky ones! I knew he was absolutely right. Our experience had been testing, it had been draining, it had been terrifying. But it seemed that our experience was over, and still my daughter was sitting in her car seat in the back of the car that very second, healthy, strong and vocal, with a future ahead of her. No measure could assess the scale of our luck, no prayer offer sufficient thanks to God, no e-mail or card express our gratitude to our friends and family, to Ian, to Michael, to the first homeopath, to Ravi; to all who had helped and supported us through what had been a truly ghastly, dark time. But now we were through. We were back in the sunshine, and aware as I'd never been before of how precious and uncertain that time spent in the sunshine is, I resolved to enjoy every scrap of it.

After that visit, I knew I had to put down the great bundle of anxiety I'd been carrying on my back, like a storybook woodsman laden with logs after a hard day's work in the forest, since Florence first became ill. It was no longer required. Florence had been well for a year. To believe in her recovery meant I needed to stop living in a state of red-alert.

Even contemplating doing this felt really frightening. I'd lived that way for so long that anything else felt reckless. But it had to be done. For the sake of all of us. Florence was undeniably well again. Johnny and I had a relationship to nurture and lives of our own to lead. Jacob, who had still had a lot of attention throughout Florence's illness, would nevertheless benefit from a more relaxed mother.

The following week, I went with Johnny to see the film *Iris*. It was my first trip to the movies in over a year and a half. So with this everyday activity, we mutually declared that our crisis was over.

Chapter Nine

Social Responsibility

The Pressure to Vaccinate

Vaccination is something that most parents in Britain decide to do. A few parents may hold back from vaccination for religious reasons or because they are committed solely to a more natural approach to health. A handful might not believe in the efficacy or safety of vaccines, while still others are committed to vaccination as a policy, but unsure about a particular vaccine in the schedule, as is the case with most parents opting for single vaccines for measles, mumps and rubella. But overall, historically, Britain has been a nation committed to vaccination, for the good of individuals and the collective population. Uptake has often exceeded 90 per cent in the past 20 years.

This high turnout is not in response to a compulsory vaccination programme, as in America. So what is it that gets parents to the surgery door? A strong sense that as a responsible and socially aware parent, you vaccinate, for the good of your child and for society at large. This feeling, or social conscience, underpins the herd immunity theory, which means that if enough children are vaccinated – usually around 95 per cent – then the disease does not have sufficient population to circulate.

We immunise to protect our own children, but also to protect others. Herd immunity ensures that those with a supressed immune system, who can't have some vaccination themselves, are still protected from the diseases, like measles, that to them could be fatal. Rubella is a vaccine done entirely to protect others – pregnant women.

This is undoubtedly a socially responsible step to take, but it does also mean that our children are subjected to more vaccines than they need to keep themselves well. It is this social responsibility theory that rules out the possibility of reducing the childhood vaccination schedule to just those that pose a serious threat, as outlined in Chapter 5.

But how far should this notion of vaccination for the greater good be extended, as more vaccines, against less and less serious conditions (one against ear infections has recently been suggested), may be added to the existing schedule?

It's not, after all, a World War situation. When my daughter Florence was ill, I didn't draw any comfort from thinking of the greater good I was bringing to the world, by ensuring that meningitis C didn't have enough of a population to circulate on, and never mind the individual consequences.

I didn't think that I was playing my small and patriotic part in liberating the world from a killer disease, whatever the personal price. I was instead crushed by the knowledge that by my having given Florence a particular vaccine, she was now seriously unwell, unwell enough for me to fear she was never going to be the same child again.

Following Florence's experience, it seems to me that my responsibility to the citizens of the UK has been replaced by a greater responsibility to my child, and to my immediate family, following a clear indication that my children have a problem with vaccination. It is on those grounds that I'm no longer prepared to send my children over the top of the trenches for the benefit of the entire nation.

I am well aware that if every mother took my viewpoint, (but thankfully not every mother had my experience) herd immunity levels would crash, and diseases we can barely remember might put in a reappearance.

Nor do I think, 'Phew, the threat of a vaccine side effect is something I can leave others to worry about.' Because obviously the threat of disease is still out there. Every time Florence is digging about in the soil planting bulbs, or falls off her bike and cuts her hand, I am conscious that her booster for tetanus is overdue, and that is because I have *made the choice for her*, that she shall not have it. The concern that many parents feel for their children's health immediately prior to and post vaccination hasn't gone away – it just, in my case, has a different flavour. The flavour of squaring up to the risk posed by the actual disease, as opposed to that of the vaccine.

This is not something it is easy to hide from. Every time a newspaper reports an imminent measles epidemic, or reports that the nation may be advised to have smallpox vaccines as we face up to the threat of germ warfare, my first thought is, what shall I do about Flo?

Vaccines and disease feature high in the news. If it's not a whooping cough outbreak, it's the recurrence of TB. All these Florence must currently face unprotected.

I would much rather be where I was before Florence's illness – able to inoculate my children against disease, 99.9 per cent certain that they would be fine. So is there anything that could bring parents like me back to vaccination?

Identifying the at-risk group

Some kind of screening system to identify those children most at risk from a particular vaccine would be a big step in the right direction. It could significantly reduce the number of severe reactions, as well as quite possibly enabling parents like me, who have already witnessed the dark side of vaccination, to consider giving their child at least the most critical vaccines. There are, after all, several types of vaccines, and a reaction against one type does not guarantee a reaction against another.

The idea that some people can take vaccination, and others can't, has been around for some time. When Wakefield sounded the alarm about the MMR, he didn't suggest that the MMR was causing autism in all children, rather that to a (growing) minority group it proved too much for their immune systems to deal with.

This notion is backed up by the experience of the parent support group Justice Awareness and Basic Support (JABS), who say on their website:

> We currently have 1800 children registered with JABS believed to have been severely affected by childhood vaccines. About two thirds of the families who have completed questionnaires report a family history of allergies, for example, asthma, hayfever, antibiotics, etc. and/or a family history of immune system problems like diabetes, arthritis, epilepsy, Crohn's disease etc. What we suspect ... is that if a child has inherited a sensitive immune system then he/she may not cope as well with a vaccine virus.

Following Florence's experience, I began to investigate my own family history. I have a father with asthma, and I have mild but persistent eczema that recurs a few times a year in the obvious places: elbows, behind the knees, in between my fingers. I have a brother with Crohn's disease, and another primary relative has epilepsy. Florence now has asthma, but this may be a small legacy of her battle with the meningitis C vaccine. Jacob has eczema. Both had a febrile convulsion prior to Florence's illness – Jacob aged three, Florence when she was one; a family tendency towards febrile convulsions is another trait that may indicate a child who will react badly to vaccination.

We certainly fit the JABS criteria. And as one scientist put it when I regaled him with my family history, 'Well, your immune system is truly messed up.' The recommendation was that I approach further vaccination for Florence with extreme caution. It may not be a medical diagnosis, but I am taking his warning seriously. As things stand at the moment, there is no alternative.

Immunity testing

There is one tool that already exists – unfortunately only privately for those who can pay – that's useful for parents in my situation. Immunity testing can tell a parent the precise state of their child's immunity. It can also save parents from giving their children unnecessary jabs.

'Boosters' of live vaccines are given routinely. The MMR is an example. The second MMR jab, given when children are four, is a repeat of the original injection, intended to catch the 5 to 10 per cent of children who, the NHS estimate, didn't react to the first shot. Most children will have reacted, and will therefore already have immunity to these diseases, possibly for life, and certainly for up to 20 years. This means that the second MMR is given on a purely speculative basis to all children of a certain age, and is unnecessary for at least 90 per cent of them.

Immunity testing can prevent this. A blood test can reveal the level of immunity a child has against measles, mumps and rubella. If the original vaccine 'took', there is clearly no benefit to their having a second shot. This theory can be applied to other vaccines as well.

Vaccination in the 21ˢᵗ century

As microbiology and its developments surge ahead, what is the future for vaccination? It may transpire that we have barely begun to explore the potential of this tool. Certainly as science marches on, waging its war against the menacing armies of disease, investigating the possibility of vaccines to protect against a wide range of conditions on the basis that prevention is much easier than cure, there is a possibility that vaccination is a medical tool still in its infancy.

There is much talk of a range of vaccines for a variety of cancers. A cervical cancer vaccine may become routine for girls within five years, for example. Vaccines against syphillis, ulcers, Parkinson's disease, Alzheimer's, and osteoporosis are all under development, and that's only naming a few.

Everyone can imagine the relief that such vaccines would bring. There can hardly be a family in the land who remains untouched by the havoc cancer can wreak. To be free of the fear of it, as much as the reality, would be extraordinary. Similarly, osteoporosis affects many post-menopausal women, curtailing their physical abilities, while Parkinson's and Alzheimer's can reduce the most intellectually able person to a confused and forgetful individual that is possibly a danger to themselves.

Many of these vaccines would be therapeutic, given when the patient was already suffering from the condition. Others under development include vaccines for arthritis, multiple sclerosis, malaria, high cholesterol and hayfever.

Vaccines to help tackle addictions like nicotine and cocaine are also in the pipeline, with the intention being to help former users from relapsing. A nicotine vaccine would take away the 'kick' that smokers get from a cigarette. A vaccine against cocaine would prevent a user from feeling the cocaine high.

Research is ongoing into new methods of delivery. One of the criticisms of vaccination is that needles are so unpleasant. If an alternative route were found, it's thought that aversion to vaccination would decline.

Meanwhile, genetic mapping is advancing by the day, giving away more and more about the way the body works. This has a knock-on effect with the development of vaccination, but we are still a considerable number of years away from this changing the face of vaccination.

Still, all steps taking us closer to that disease-free Utopia, we might think.

But, before we walk this road, shouldn't we ask one question? Is vaccination truly such a magical tool, a perfect cure-all? From a medic's point of view, prevention may be far easier than cure, but equally, in the past and present, the dream of protection against disease, has, for some parents and children, undoubtedly become a nightmare. There is no reason to expect that any new vaccines will not present the drawbacks that the current ones do. So while the prospect of a vaccine against absolutely everything might seem marvellous to some, shouldn't this perceived benefit be balanced against the risk posed by the agent being vaccinated against?

Obviously this is easier to do with therapeutic vaccination. After all, the patient does not have seemingly perfect health at stake. But for those that do – and that includes the majority of children vaccinated – the reality is that just because it is possible to create a vaccine against almost everything, doesn't mean parents automatically want to give them to their children.

The intrinsic problem with seeing all disease, dangerous and mild, as something to be eradicated at all costs, is that we may be in danger of losing something our children need – a practice round in the ring for their developing immune systems.

The 'hygiene hypothesis' is a theory which suggests that over-zealous cleaning of houses has meant immune systems lack practice fighting bacteria and viruses. This means that when people do come into contact with an allergen, the immune system does not destroy it as it should. The result can be something like asthma – against which, in a rather terrifying full circle, a vaccine is now being developed to combat the meteoric rise in cases.

Dr Ratko Djukanovic of the University of Southampton, who is leading research into an asthma vaccine, told BBC News, October 2001:

> This vaccine is based on the idea that we live in an environment that is too clean. We have changed the balance of the environment and our bodies have become over-protected through the use of antibiotics, vaccination programmes and cleanliness.
>
> If we protect children too much from the environment, then their immune system does not learn to respond in a balanced manner.

Are we over-protecting our children by vaccinating them against such a wide range of diseases? If, as some medics and alternative practitioners seem to be saying, far from posing a threat to our children, some diseases actually lead to better long-term health, why are we still so focused on fighting to prevent them occurring at all?

Is it possible that we have reached the stage in our society when every disease must be anticipated and suppressed, in order to enable us to live our busy lives uninterrupted by the call to nurse a sick child for a few days? If this is so, how much of this is a result of the culture of long working hours that many parents may have, or are expected to have, today? Have we simply reached a position when there is just no time for children to be sick, because if they are, the creche or school won't take them and someone has to interrupt a busy life to look after them, to the detriment of their employment? Not to mention the billions of pounds companies lose through absent workers.

Certainly in America it has been suggested that the primary reason for inoculating children with varicella vaccine is to stop parents losing days at work. One study estimated that parents lost between 0.5 and 1.8 work days to caring for a child with chickenpox. Taken across America, this is a huge number of work days 'saved' in economic terms. In 'The Vaccine Guide' by Randall Neustaedter (from which the lost work days figures also come), it is claimed that 'Vaccination of the entire population will save an estimated $380 million in lost income and wages.' By inoculating the entire child population, many of these 'lost' days could be prevented.

But at what cost to the child? In addition to the issue of the unnecessary increase in their vaccine load, there is also no certainty that this vaccine does not wane with time. Introduced in 1995, will America soon find itself with a generation of young adults with no immunity to chickenpox? In adults the disease is not the mild experience it generally is in children. A great many more work days may very well be lost in the future, as a result of this mass experiment. How much more sensible to allow children to have chickenpox as children, when the disease is mild, and receive the benefit of lifelong immunity?

If children need to be allowed to be sick with the minor common childhood ailments for their long-term good, we clearly have to structure their home lives and our greater society in a way that enables this fundamental process of development to occur. The alternative – of subjecting our children to a range of vaccines that we know they are better off without and that might also actively cause them some damage, to enable our lives to carry on at a speed and profitability that has become the norm – is unthinkable.

Long-term trials

There is no certainty that vaccination does not have long-term implications on health. My generation is a living trial for the many vaccines that we were given, 30 years on. Yet little or no research is being done into the state of health of that generation, and therefore nothing learned. Impressionistically, we know that we generally live longer than previous generations, but we should not be complacent. Once again the long-term effects of vaccination have been questioned – does childhood vaccination, for example, cause some to develop multiple sclerosis, or arthritis, or cancer, decades later? No answers are forthcoming. Long-term trials might help to provide some.

We don't have such trials and quite clearly we should. In order to draw maximum understanding of vaccination, and the side effects of vaccines, precise records of every vaccine a person has in their lifetime should be recorded. To do this successfully, we need to get beyond the everyday muddle of lost medical records, which leave no ability to trace whether an illness could possibly be related to a vaccine given long ago.

Dr Jefferson, co-ordinator of the Cochrane Collaboration's vaccine research, an organisation dedicated to providing independent scientific research, believes technology has the answer to this particular problem. If the public could get over their aversion to the notion of identity cards (and there is obviously a civil rights issue here), these cards could be used to record such information. Immunisation registers could be created, making it incredibly easy to run long-term trials on the effects of various vaccines. Patients could be monitored over decades. He said: 'Vaccination registers would be one way to achieve this. Half the battle would be won, as we would know who has been exposed to what. The idea is to have a cohort which we can interrogate retrospectively. We may start making good inferences.'

A vaccination library

Dr Jefferson also has a dream. He believes there is a place for an independent international database library, that brings together all the available evidence in existence on vaccination: information gleaned from past trials and from research into vaccines of all kinds. The advantage of this on-line library would be its availablity to everyone – scientists and vaccine consumers.

Parents – like those currently confused by the ongoing MMR crisis – would be able to search for information on any vaccine they were concerned about. With all the information literally at their fingertips, they would be better placed than they have ever been to make as informed a decision for their child as possible. As would travellers contemplating shots before going abroad, or a cancer patient being offered a therapeutic vaccination for his condition.

On a professional basis, researchers carrying out a review of a type of vaccine would be able to access all past work on the subject, together with interviews with the original scientists who carried out the work. This kind of information resource, such a simple but necessary idea, simply doesn't exist at present.

Dr Jefferson said: 'This library has to be for the user. For the small children, the weakest members of our society, who must be looked after. That principle has to apply. If trials are carried out experimenting on human beings as young as two months, you can't just walk away.'

Vaccine safety

There may be a slow, growing awareness that vaccine safety is not as good as it could and should be. The European Union published a report recently, co-signed by Sir Michael Rawlins, chairman of the UK's National Institute for Clinical Excellence (NICE), saying that vaccine vigilance was a methodological problem. In other words, safety criteria are just not good enough.

A recent report by the EUVAX (Scientific and Technical Evaluation of Vaccination Programmes in the European Union) project discovered that the number of full-time employees working on vaccine safety in Germany, Finland and the Netherlands was just one. In Belgium, Austria, Switzerland, Denmark, Spain, Greece, Italy and Great Britain, the outcome was even worse: no single person worked full time on vaccine safety in any of these countries. The report recommended that strategic plans should be drafted for the development of national vaccinovigilance activities.

Clearly, although there may be a reluctance to address vaccination safety issues at national level, some work on the area is being done at European level, and the hope must be that eventually junior British citizens will benefit from this.

Reporting of adverse reactions

One of the ways the EUVAX report highlighted as improving vaccinovigilance was through improved reporting of adverse reactions. The key way this is done in the UK at present is through the Yellow Card system, which exists for reporting suspected adverse reactions to any medication. But one estimate of how many reactions get reported via this system reveals a depressing figure of around just 20 per cent.

Yellow cards are filled out by health workers, on the basis that the Committee on Safety of Medicines and the Medical Controls Agency, who receive them and analyse the data they provide, consider it 'vital to have your doctor's or pharmacist's interpretation of the suspected reaction in order for us to be able to evaluate the report fully'. This may work well if the doctor is in agreement with the patient about the possible link between a drug or vaccine and an adverse reaction. But what if the doctor and the patient are at odds on the issue? Florence's experiences, for example, never made it on to a yellow card.

However passionately I feel that her illness was brought about by the meningitis C vaccine, that view isn't going to go anywhere where some good might come of it. I lost count of the number of times the very idea that Florence's illness was caused by her vaccination was dismissed by a medic out of hand. I have learned from speaking to other mothers with similar experiences to mine that this is a common occurrence. For some unfathomable reason, vaccine damage is not something doctors are keen to acknowledge.

America has a reporting system that exists solely for vaccine reactions, the Vaccine Adverse Events Reporting System (VAERS) and this, in contrast to the UK's Yellow Card system, does allow anyone to complete a form, 'to ensure that all relevant data is captured'.

Couldn't Britain's parents benefit from a similar system? This would give them a voice in an important area, and although they may not be medically qualified, they are generally the people with the greatest understanding of the state of their children's health, and of any dramatic changes. They know their child in an in-depth way from being with them everyday. By dismissing their experience just because they don't have the medical background against which to set it, we may very well be throwing away critical information that could contribute to making vaccinations safer for everyone.

Chapter Ten

Taking Back Responsibility for My Children's Health

S ince Jenner's first vaccine was made compulsory, parents have been encouraged to let the state effectively make major health decisions for their children. While we agonise over many aspects of our childrearing before making our independent and varying decisions, we have, for over a century, allowed the government to dictate fundamental health choices for our offspring.

As a result of Florence's experience I was forced to wake up to the fact that the responsibility for my childrens' health lies not with the government, but with me. The NHS, and the government's recommended vaccination schedule, do not magically hold the power to protect my children against a range of frightening-sounding diseases. A vaccine doesn't come with a guarantee. It's not a case of one size fits all. Vaccination is an area that requires thought, undertaken by me, looking at my children as individuals all the while.

The result of this shift in my thinking is that I am no longer abiding by a routine vaccination schedule designed for the nation's children. Instead I have tried to determine what is the best way to keep Jacob and Florence well, with as much medical help as I can access.

Immunity testing provided me with a profile of the immunisation status of both children, which put me in the full picture. I took Jacob and Florence to a London-based paediatrician who runs a clinic offering single jabs for measles, mumps and rubella. I explained our history, and asked him to arrange for Jacob and Florence to have their immunity checked for all the childhood diseases they were immunised against as babies, given before Florence's experience challenged my thinking. He did so, agreeing that this was the most appropriate way to proceed in a situation like ours.

The results came a few days later. Despite Jacob being over two years late for his school booster, his immunity levels to measles, mumps and rubella are well above required levels. The same holds true for Florence. This essentially means I don't have to worry any more whether to give them a measles vaccine. (Since I lived until recently in an area that apparently has an MMR uptake of just 60 per cent, this gave me huge peace of mind.)

However, both Jacob's and Florence's immunity to diptheria, tetanus, pertussis is lower than considered sufficient to ward off the diseases. Jacob has immunity to polio, but Florence does not. This latter result is an interesting example of the variables of vaccination. Jacob received his last polio immunisation six years ago, while Florence had hers just four and a half years ago. Yet it is Jacob who remains immune, and not Florence. Is this discrepency down to the batch they had, or a result of the way they individually metabolise the vaccine? No one can tell. What it certainly is an example of is how we all react differently to vaccination.

What the immunity test also tells me is that if I want to maintain Jacob's immunity as recommended by the NHS, he needs a tetanus jab, plus diptheria and pertussis. Florence needs all this as well as polio.

Tetanus and polio vaccines apparently carry a very low risk of side effects. They are also diseases that everyone I have interviewed for this book has pinpointed as being vaccines worth having. So I feel I should give them to Jacob. He, after all, doesn't have Florence's vaccination history. But when I discover that the single tetanus jab contains thimerosal, it seems an impossible step to take.

If I can find him a thimerosal-free tetanus vaccine, I will seriously consider giving it to him. He is forever falling over in the school playground, and coming back with deep cuts in his hand. If the safest possible tetanus vaccine were available to him, Jacob should very probably have it.

With Florence, the situation is obviously much more difficult. However much I would like to give her protection against these diseases, without any way of knowing how she will react to it, my mind stalls at the thought.

It seems we have only recently returned from the shadowy land of extreme ill-health, where the prevailing emotions are fear and exhaustion. Even now, now that Florence is generally considered well, she bears the slight scars of her experience. She is asthmatic, something that dates from the battle with pneumonia, and very vulnerable to chest infections. How could we even begin to consider giving her something that just might take her there again?

We can't. Instead, we will continue to focus on other preventive health measures, starting with good nutrition. We will carry on visiting our homeopath every three months, and continue to visit Michael, our cranial osteopath, every now and then as well. Until science has something else to offer, this currently seems my best course of action for keeping my children well.

NOT A DAY passes when I don't feel grateful for the family life I have. I know, from talking to mothers whose children have experienced much more severe cases of vaccine damage than mine, how very differently it could have turned out. While my life has reverted to normal, they carry on each day, battling to get the best help and support for their children, in far from easy circumstances.

That doesn't mean I'm over it all together. While our family life now moves in normal waters, I find it hard to banish from my mind a story I heard, of another child who had a bad reaction to the meningitis C vaccine and recovered, only to relapse about two years later. Of course this chills my blood momentarily, but I can't let Florence's life – or mine – be run by fear. She is currently a normal, healthy, happy girl of four and a half, and all I can do is hope and pray she stays that way.

Life serves to remind me at every turn just how fortunate I am. I read a snippet in *The Times* not long ago, which detailed how sodium valporate had been responsible for the deaths of several small children. This was the same drug a paediatric neurololgist had recommended for Florence – a drug which Johnny and I eventually decided not to put her on. Similarly, flicking through the Sunday papers the other day, I came across an article written by a girl in her early twenties, who developed epilepsy as a teenageer – something doctors put down to a febrile convulsion she had when she was 18 months old.

Who knows what the future holds for Florence? (But then who knows what it holds for any of us?) I focus on the fact that it is over two years since she last had a convulsion. Since then, she has had the occasional temperature which has passed without incident. While the temperature lasts and my suppressed fears bloom into panic, I force myself to remember what Ravi said to me two years ago, in his soft voice filled with smiles: 'You don't have to worry about convulsions anymore.'

I believe Ravi's right. I feel the benefits of my luck every day. But I also expect that I will stop worrying about Flo when she's, oh, fifty? Such is the almost imperceptible emotional limp with which I walk, a residue from those anxious, frankly terrible, days. But I recognise that it is a very small price to pay, and I pay it willingly.